Reproductive Wellness
Acupuncture & Integrative Medicine

The Secret to Conception

Teaching The Womb

Workbook

Sage de Beixedon Breslin, Ph.D

Marc Sklar, L.Ac, FABORM

The Secret to Conception: Teaching The Womb
Workbook
Copyright © 2014 Sage de Beixedon Breslin, Ph.D.
& Marc Sklar, L.Ac, FABORM
All Rights Reserved
ISBN-10: 1499390416
ISBN-13: 978-1499390414

This document is copyrighted and posted
with permission by Reproductive Wellness, Inc..
While you are welcome to utilize these materials for yourself, the founders of Reproductive Wellness, Inc. ask that all others purchase the *Secret to Conception Workbook* from http://www.reproductivewellness.com/.

Reading about strategies to improve your fertility is a great start, but the secret to reproductive success lies in emotional and behavioral change. Within these pages are a wide variety of strategies and interventions to *practice,* so that your dreams become reality!

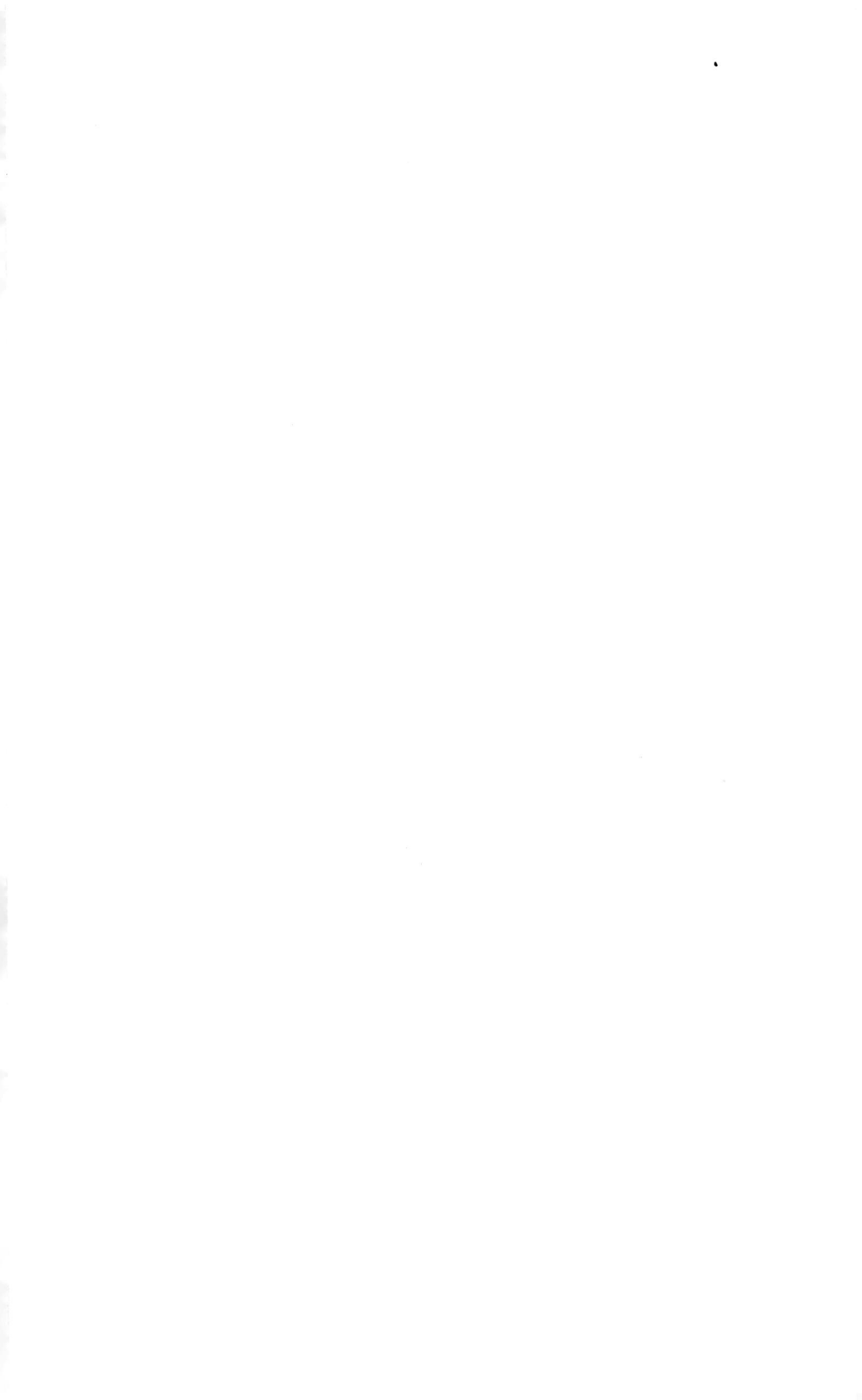

Table of Contents

Chapter 1: Fertility Questionnaire: Identifying Fertility Challenges & Factors — 1

Chapter 2: Fertility Organizational Chart: Who's on your Fertility Team? — 11

Chapter 3: What's in Your Head? Beliefs, Ideas & Historical Messages to which you've been Exposed — 13

Chapter 4: Family Values Questionnaire: What's Important? — 23

Chapter 5: Infertility Factors: Male, Female, Couple, & Unexplained Infertility — 27

Chapter 6: Stress Scale — 35

Chapter 7: Stress Map — 37

Chapter 8: Body Mapping — 41

Chapter 9: Stress-Inducing Self-Talk — 45

Chapter 10: Stress-Reducing Self-Talk — 51

Chapter 11: Nutrition: What are You Eating, or What's Eating You? — 55

Recipes — 73

Power Pilaf — 75

Black Bean, Corn and Tomato Salad — 77

Quick Chicken Tostadas	79
Baked Mahi-Mahi	81
Black Bean and Pumpkin Soup	83
Santa Fe Bean Mashers	85
Skillet Chili	87
Making a plan of Action	89
Chapter 12: Relaxation Exercises	93
Chapter 13: Yoga : Postures for Optimal Health & Fertility	107
Chapter 14: Guided Imagery	133
Chapter 15: Cognitive Concepts for Conception	147
Chapter 16: Fertility & Feelings	159
Chapter 17: Listening to your Lover	173
Chapter 18: Old Baggage I Carry	195
Chapter 19: Commitment to Love: Agreement for the NOW, as well as for the Future	199
Chapter 20: Resources for Family Alternatives	205

Chapter 1: Fertility Questionnaire: Identifying Fertility Challenges & Factors

Name:_____
_____

Date: _____

| **Menstrual History** |

1. Age at which your menstruation began _____
2. (Please circle one) Are your periods: Like clockwork / Somewhat regular / Erratic
3. What is the interval between your menstrual cycles? _____ days.
4. If your period is erratic, please complete the following statement: My period always comes sometime between _____ days and _____ days after the completion of my previous cycle.

5. During a typical menstrual period, how many days of bleeding do you have? _____

6. (Please circle one) Is your bleeding: Light / Normal / Heavy

7. Which of the following describes the predominant color of your menstrual blood? (Please circle)

   Light Red   Bright Red   Dark Red   Purple
   Brown   Black

8. Is there clotting with your period?   Yes / No

9. Do you regularly experience PMS?   Yes / No (Circle which symptoms best describe your PMS)

   Breast tenderness or swelling / Irritability Abdominal Bloating / Diarrhea / Constipation Pain and Cramping / Headaches or Migraines Mood Swings / Low Back Pain / Dizziness Extreme Fatigue / Acne / Food Cravings

10. During your menstrual flow, how many times would you soak a tampon or pad in a 4 hour time?_____

11. On what day of your cycle do you ovulate? _____

12. During ovulation, is your cervical mucus clear, abundant and stretchy? If not, please describe._____
    _____

13. What is the most important thing that you think your acupuncturist should know about your menstrual cycle?
    _____

14. Have you had a venereal disease?   Yes / No

If yes, please describe:

_____

15. Do you have a history with any of the following:

    Regularly occurring yeast infections ... Yes / No

    An abnormal pap smear .... Yes / No

    Any kind of uterine surgery .... Yes / No

    Endometriosis .... Yes / No

    Chronic vaginal discharge .... Yes / No

    Uterine fibroids or polyps .... Yes / No

    Pelvis Inflammatory Disease .... Yes / No

    Polycystic ovarian syndrome .... Yes / No

    Spotting or bleeding between periods. Yes / No

16. Have you used oral contraceptives? .... Yes / No

    If yes, please list the dates of use, and disuse below:

    _____
    _____
    _____
    _____

Fertility History

1. Have you ever been pregnant before? ..... Yes / No

3

Total number of pregnancies: _____

Number of vaginal deliveries: _____

Number of Cesarian (c-section) deliveries: _____

Number of Abortions: _____

Number of Miscarriages: _____

Number of still births: _____

If you have ever had a miscarriage, please list the week of pregnancy when the miscarriage occurred and the reason (if known):
_____

2. During ovulation do you experience the following:

    Pain or cramping .... Yes / No

    Bleeding or spotting .... Yes / No

    Copious or excessive discharge .... Yes / No

    Breast pain or tenderness .... Yes / No

3. During ovulation is your cervical mucous (circle one)

    Clear/stretchy   Dense/cloudy   Unknown

4. How long have you been actively trying to get pregnant?
_____

5. Do you have a committed partner with whom you are trying to conceive? Yes / No

6. How long have you been married/ living together?_____

7. Has he had a male fertility work-up? Yes / No

   If yes, what were the results? _____

   If no, do you intend to get one? Yes / No

8. Have you ever undergone fertility treatments or used Assisted Repro. Technology?

   Yes / No

   If yes, please describe the methods that you have used and the dates for each procedure:

   _____
   _____
   _____
   _____

9. Have you ever taken medication to help you ovulate? Yes / No

   If yes, when? and for how long?
   _____

10. Have your fallopian tubes been evaluated medically? Yes / No

11. What were the results
    _____

12. Have you had any hormonal lab tests done?

    What were the results?
    _____

13. Have you been given any biomedical diagnosis that might explain why you are having trouble getting pregnant? Yes / No

14. Have you ever charted your Basal Body Temperature (BBT) Yes / No

    If yes, please bring your charts to your next appointment.

15. Disregarding anything that anyone has told you previously, why do YOU think that you are having difficulty getting pregnant?

    _____

16. On a one to ten scale, how would you rate your commitment level to doing whatever it takes to getting pregnant? (Including making dietary and lifestyle changes / quitting smoking and drinking alcohol / taking herbs regularly) _____

Health History

Kidney

Do you have vaginal Dryness ☐ Y ☐ N

Is your midcycle cervical mucus scanty or missing?
☐ Y ☐ N

Does your menstrual blood tend to be dull in color?
☐ Y ☐ N

Do you feel cold cramps during your period that responds to heat?
☐ Y ☐ N

Spleen

Is your menstruation thin, watery, profuse, or pink in color?
☐ Y ☐ N

Are you more tired around ovulation or menstruation?
☐ Y ☐ N

Have you ever been diagnosed with uterine prolapse?
☐ Y ☐ N

Are your menstrual cramps accompanied by a bearing-down sensation in your uterus?   ☐ Y ☐ N

Blood

Are your menses scanty and/or late?
☐ Y ☐ N

Is your menstrual flow ever brown or black in color?
☐ Y ☐ N

Do you have painful, unmovable breast lumps?
☐ Y ☐ N

Can you feel any abnormal lumps in your lower abdomen?
☐ Y ☐ N

Do you have piercing or stabbing menstrual cramps?
☐ Y ☐ N

Liver

Do you feel bloated or irritable around ovulation?

☐ Y ☐ N

Does it feel as if your ovulation lasts longer than it should?

☐ Y ☐ N

Do you experience nipple pain or discharge from your nipples?

☐ Y ☐ N

Have you been diagnosed with elevated prolactin levels?

☐ Y ☐ N

Are your menses painful? ☐ Y ☐ N

Do you feel your menstrual cramps in the external genital area?

☐ Y ☐ N

Is the menstrual blood thick and dark, or purplish in color?

☐ Y ☐ N

Damp

Do you break out with red acne (especially premenstrually)?

☐ Y ☐ N

Do you have a short menstrual cycle? ☐ Y ☐ N

Do you have vaginal irritation or rashes? ☐ Y ☐ N

Do you have fibrocystic breasts? ☐ Y ☐ N

Do you have cystic or pustular acne? ☐ Y ☐ N

Do you have foul smelling, yellow or greenish vaginal discharge?

☐ Y ☐ N

Are you prone to vaginal and/or rectal itching during your luteal or premenstrual phase? ☐ Y ☐ N

Chapter 2: Fertility Organizational Chart: Who's on your Fertility Team?

Our team members include clinicians from the fields of Health Psychology, Traditional Chinese Medicine, Acupuncture, Herbal Medicine, Nutrition, and Wellness and Exercise.

Who would you add to your Integrative Medical Team?

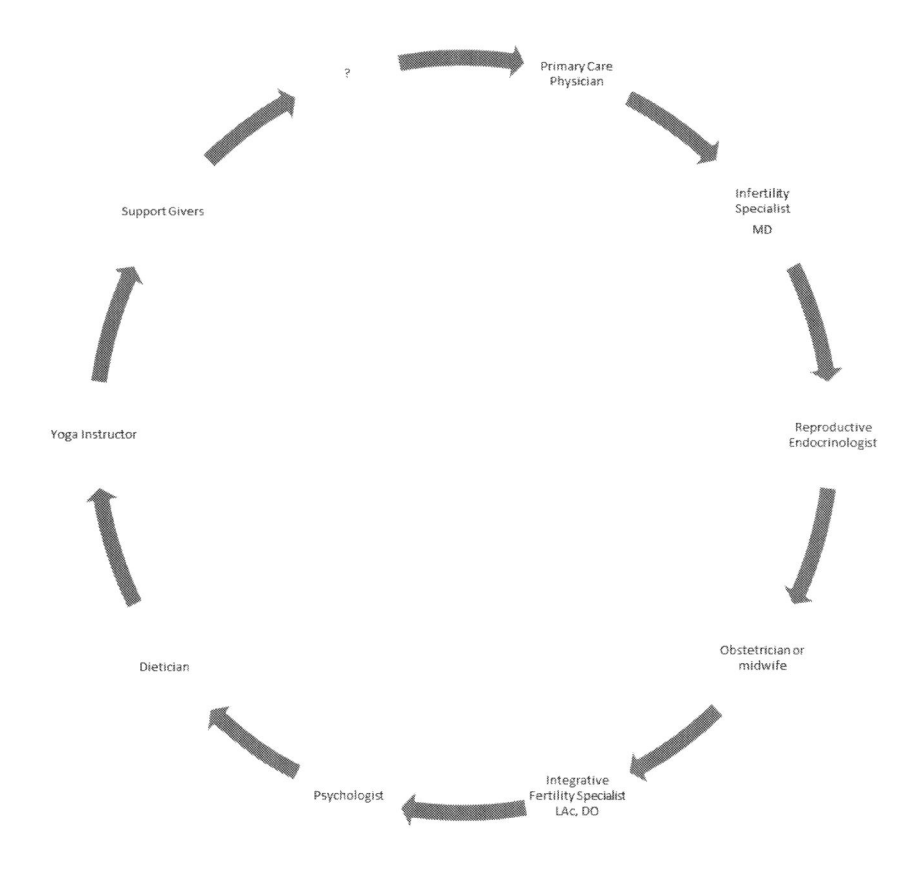

```
                    ?  ──→  Primary Care
                              Physician
                                  │
                                  ↓
   Support Givers            Infertility
       ↑                      Specialist
       │                          MD
                                  │
                                  ↓
   Yoga Instructor           Reproductive
       ↑                     Endocrinologist
       │                          │
                                  ↓
     Dietician               Obstetrician or
       ↑                        midwife
       │                          │
                                  ↓
              Psychologist  ←  Integrative
                               Fertility Specialist
                                  LAc, DO
```

Chapter 3: What's in Your Head?: Beliefs, Ideas & Historical Messages to which you've been Exposed

What are your beliefs?

- About yourself?

- Are you a good person?

  _____
  _____
  _____
  _____
  _____

Do you deserve to have a healthy relationship?

_____

_____

_____

_____

_____

Do you deserve to have a family?

_____

_____

_____

_____

_____

Do children come naturally?

_____

_____

_____

_____

_____

_____

Are there things that stand in your way of what you want?

- What are they?

  _____
  _____
  _____
  _____
  _____
  _____

- About your partner?

Is your partner a good person?

  _____
  _____
  _____
  _____
  _____
  _____

Does your partner love you?

  _____
  _____
  _____

Is your partner equally committed to this process in order to achieve life change, as well as pregnancy?

Does your partner blame or resent you for the challenges with fertility?

Is your partner in it for the long haul?

_____

_____

- About your partnership or marriage?

    Is your partnership or marriage strong enough to endure the challenges of this process?

    _____
    _____
    _____
    _____

    _____

    Will your partnership or marriage survive even if you are unable to conceive?

    _____
    _____
    _____
    _____

    _____

    Is this relationship the right one for you?

    _____
    _____

_____

_____

_____

- About life?

Life is fair / not fair?

_____

_____

_____

_____

_____

Life is easy / hard?

_____

_____

_____

_____

_____

Challenges can / cannot be overcome?

_____

_____

_____

_____

People are there to help / hurt?

_____

Good people do / do not exist in the world?

_____

The world is / is not safe for you to bring children into?

- About pregnancy?

Can every woman become pregnant?

_____
_____
_____
_____

_____

Is there some physical, emotional, relational or cultural reason why you cannot become pregnant?

_____
_____
_____
_____

_____

Is pregnancy "right" for you?

_____
_____
_____
_____

_____

Can you revere the pregnant form?

_____
_____
_____
_____

_____

Will you be able to become pregnant and deliver a healthy baby?

_____
_____
_____
_____

_____

Are you caught in any gender traps?

Infertility is primarily a woman's problem

Women are the only ones who need to be involved in the solution (eg. fertility treatments and interventions).

Men are not supposed to show their feelings, even if failing to do so inhibits conception.

_____
_____

_____

_____

_____

_____

_____

_____

- What are some of the gender traps at work in your world?

_____

_____

_____

_____

_____

The responses to all of these questions impact how you think and feel about yourself, your partner, your relationship, and your fertility. Careful consideration must be made of your responses.

Do they enable you to move forward or are they inhibiting your progress towards connection and conception?

Chapter 4: Family Values Questionnaire: What's Important?

The values that you and your partner hold may greatly impact your health, wellness and fertility.

Consider the following values and determine which of the values enhance your fertility and which values may actually inhibit your fertility. Use a red pen to outline or highlight those values that may inhibit growth in your relationship or may not promote conception. Use a green pen or highlighter to identify those values which enhance your relationship and your potential for conception and healthy pregnancy. Both you, and your partner, can complete the questionnaire, then share the results!

- Achievement - Accomplishment, results brought about by persistence
- Advancement - Opportunity to make rapid moves upward in a hierarchy.
- Adventure - Excitement, action, fast pace, taking risks in a business sense

- Affiliation - Having close relationships with others; cooperation; friendship.
- Autonomy - Doing things on my own, without having a lot of rules, orders or directions.
- Balance - Sufficient time for pursuits outside of work; for balance between work and personal/family life.
- Community - Involvement in community affairs and activities.
- Creativity - Opportunity to express my own ideas, continually living in new and untested ways.
- Decisions/Power - Having the power to decide a course of action, direction, policies; being the one in charge.
- Economic security - Able to count on economic resources; freedom from money worries.
- Emotional well-being - Peace of mind, quickly resolving inner conflicts.
- Help Society - Doing something that contributes to the betterment of the world or community where I live; serving a cause.
- High earning - Monetary rewards or the potential for increased monetary rewards in the future.
- Honesty/Authenticity - Being frank and genuinely yourself with others and having them be that way with you.
- Humor/Fun - Freedom to be spontaneous, playful, humorous, having laughs; keeping things in a lighter perspective
- Independence - Doing things by myself, without lots of contact with other people; solitude.

- Influence people - Be in a position to change attitudes or actions of other people; leading through knowledge or expertise
- Intellectual Challenge - Learning new things, stimulating the mind.
- Justice/Fairness - Treating others impartially, wanting equity for others and myself.
- Location - Living in a place (town, geographical area) that is conducive to my lifestyle and things I enjoy doing.
- Love/Family - Affection, intimacy, caring, attachment to a family.
- Physical challenge - Meeting physical demands; physical risk-taking.
- Physical Environment - Clean, comfortable, pleasant space and surroundings.
- Project identity - Able to produce tangibles, seeing end results of my work.
- Recognition/Respect - Having others acknowledge me as important; prestige; public approval and acclaim; people look up to me because of what I do.
- Religious/Spiritual Conviction - Communion with or activity on behalf of God or other higher power.
- Service - Being involved in helping other people directly, individually or in small groups.
- Stability - Certainty, slower pace of change; preferring to keep things on an even keel.
- Structure - Having a defined set of expectations from others knowing what is expected within defined rules or guidelines.

- Tranquility - Serenity; freedom from pressures and "the rat race."
- Variety - New and challenging experiences; using new resources or abilities in new situations; novelty, change.

One of the Values Inventories which is available to the general public is offered at http://www.decisionbooks.com/pdf/values1.pdf. Other resources for the exploration of values can be found at http://www.life-values.com/index.html.

Chapter 5: Infertility Factors: Male, Female, Couple, & Unexplained Infertility

a. What's Stopping You?
   i. Male Factor Infertility

   Male factor infertility refers to the inability of a man's sperm to fertilize an ovum. Male fertility depends on three primary elements:

   - there must be adequate spermatozoa production by the testes
   - the sperm must be able to travel unobstructed through the seminal duct and
   - the sperm must reach the ovum without fail.

These elements often go awry and produce the following fertility challenges:

> Low sperm count: this is defined as less than 20 million sperm per milliliter (the "normal" sperm count is 200 million per ejaculate)
> Low sperm motility: this is defined as less than 50% of the sperm have purposeful forward movement towards the ovum.
> Poor sperm morphology: this is defined as less than 30% of the sperm having normal form and shape.

What challenges, if any does the male partner in your relationship have with regards to fertility?

☐ Male partner has problems with sperm count

☐ Male partner has problems with sperm motility

☐ Male partner has problems with sperm morphology

ii. Female Factor Infertility

There are many conditions associated with female factor infertility. Some of those medical challenges include:

- ➤ Secondary Infertility
- ➤ Uterine and Pelvic Abnormalities
- ➤ Hostile Cervical Mucus
- ➤ Irregular Ovulation and
- ➤ Polycystic Ovarian Syndrome

Secondary Infertility

Secondary infertility can be caused by a wide range of issues, including age, irregular ovulation, endometriosis, hostile cervical mucus, abnormal uterus or pelvis, impact from prior birth experience, and miscarriage .

Of the issues above, are there concerns or challenges with:

- ☐ Age (older than 35 years old)
- ☐ Irregular ovulation
- ☐ History of endometriosis
- ☐ Hostile cervical mucus or "sperm allergy"

- ☐ Tipped, prolapsed or bifurcated uterus
- ☐ Abnormal pelvic area
- ☐ Scarring or other conditions subsequent to prior miscarriage or birth experience

Uterine and Pelvic Abnormalities

Issues associated with an abnormal pelvis or uterus can also create reproductive challenges.

Have you experienced any of the following conditions or concerns?

- ☐ Birth defects affecting the reproductive organs
- ☐ Uterine fibroids
- ☐ Insufficient endometrial lining
- ☐ Endometriosis in the uterus, fallopian tubes or pelvic cavity
- ☐ Disease and/or damage to the fallopian tubes
- ☐ Adhesions and/or damage to the pelvic cavity.

Hostile Cervical Mucus

Hostile cervical mucus can prevent advancement through the birth canal to the fallopian tubes.

Of the following conditions associated with hostile cervical mucus, have you experienced:

- ☐ Mucus containing antibodies to sperm ("sperm allergy")
- ☐ Excessively thick cervical mucus
- ☐ Inadequate estrogen stimulation

Irregular Ovulation

Irregular ovulation affects many women. Are you one of them?

Do you have a history of any of the patterns below with regards to your menstrual periods?

- ☐ Primary amenorrhea – lack of a first menstrual cycle
- ☐ Secondary amenorrhea – lack of menses after initial menstruation
- ☐ Polymenorrhea – more than one menstrual cycle within a 26-day period
- ☐ Hypomenorrhea – significant reduction in the length and volume of menses

Ovulatory conditions can also be subsequent to other problems and disorders. Consider the following questions:

- ☐ *Have you gone into premature menopause?*
- ☐ *Do you have Polycystic Ovarian Syndrome?*
- ☐ *Have you undergone chemotherapy?*
- ☐ *Do you have tumors in your brain or reproductive organs which might affect ovulation?*
- ☐ *Have you had or do you currently have chronic infection in your reproductive organs?*
- ☐ *Do you engage in lengthy or intense exercise?*
- ☐ *Have you had significant weight change over the last six months?*
- ☐ *Do you produce excessive levels of prolactin?*

Polycystic Ovarian Syndrome

PCOS is an extremely common metabolic disorder which can drastically affect fertility. Many women go undiagnosed until they find themselves unable to conceive. In order to recognize your own risk factors for PCOS, respond to the following questions:

- ☐ *Are you Latina, Native American or Asian?*
- ☐ *Do you have raised androgen or testosterone levels?*
- ☐ *Do you have multiple or recurrent cysts on your ovaries?*
- ☐ *Are your menses irregular (when not taking Oral Contraception)?*
- ☐ *Do you have extremely light menstrual periods?*
- ☐ *Are you overweight, even if only by 5-10% of body weight?*
- ☐ *Do you have excessive hair growth (on the face, pubic region, and abdomen particularly)*
- ☐ *Do you have acne?*
- ☐ *Have you been diagnosed with Insulin Resistance Syndrome (IR)?*
- ☐ *Have you been diagnosed with Type 2 Diabetes Mellitus?*
- ☐ *Do you have high blood pressure?*
- ☐ *Do you have high cholesterol?*
- ☐ *Do you have a history of Cardiovascular Disease?*

iii. "Unexplained" Infertility

And, after all is said and done, perhaps none of these challenges appears to explain your inability to conceive and maintain a pregnancy. Perhaps your infertility has *yet to be explained!*

Chapter 6: Stress Scale

When you consider your first attempts to conceive, how did you feel? What were your thoughts? How high was your stress level? If there were any circumstances associated with increased stress in your life, what were they? What was the end result?

Stress has been studied broadly using the Holmes and Rahe Social Readjustment Rating Scale. This inventory lists a broad range of events and transitions that can be associated with the experience of stress. Each item on the scale is assigned a value or weight. Depending on how many items you select based on your own experiences indicates how much stress your being is trying to manage.

To explore the SRRS, visit
http://www.stresstips.com/lifeevents.htm or
http://okvoices.org/stress.html

Chapter 7: Stress Map

In order to combat stress, you must be able to identify how, *and where*, it impacts your body. Some common physical signs of stress include:

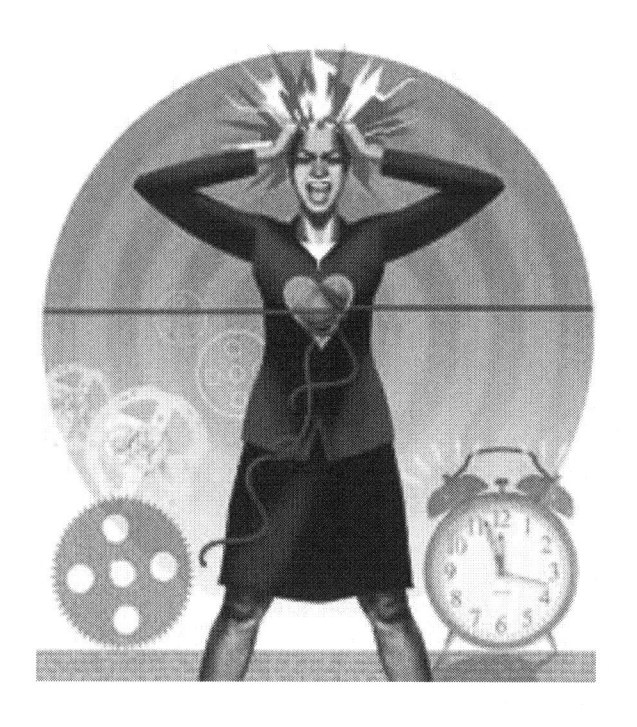

- Furrowed eyebrows
- Dilated pupils
- Tightness in the throat
- Frequent sore throat
- Tightness in shoulders
- Tense and aching neck
- Bloated stomach
- Incontinence
- Diarrhea
- Cold fingers/feet
- Clammy palms
- Rigid pelvis
- Numb genitals
- Large muscles tight
- Constricted arteries
- Fast pulse
- Shallow breathing

What does your body tell you?

_____

_____

_____

What areas of your body suggest that you might be experiencing stress?

How might this affect your ability to conceive?

Chapter 8: Body Mapping

The Chinese believe that certain emotions are stored in specific parts of the body, and that when an excess of that emotion exists there, the body experiences tension, as well as other symptoms in that part of the body.

From head to toe, those areas are:

- ➢ From the eyes to the throat, the body may harbor sadness. The typical "lump in the throat" is a sign of unexpressed sadness.
- ➢ From ear to ear at the jawline, the body may hold happiness and joy. Ever been so happy that you just beamed incessantly, then experienced tightness in your jaw or even a headache?
- ➢ Anger is experienced as a crown around the top of the skull, or as low as the temples.
- ➢ Frustration is said to live at the base of the skull, extending out across the shoulders.

- The "weight of the world" is said to be held between the shoulder blades- the "Atlas" area may ache in response to excess responsibility and financial stress.
- In the heart, the body stores the ecstasy, as well as the agony, of love.
- From the sternum to the intestine, the body may hold anxiety and despair. Recall those expressions "butterflies in the stomach" as well as "in the pit of my stomach".
- From the abdomen to the knees, the body holds fear. How often have you heard, "I felt weak in the knees" or "I felt as if my knees were going to give out beneath me"?
- In the lower back lives hopelessness, when one's *being* is insufficiently supported.
- And in the feet, lives the flexibility to roll with it all and still stay centered (pain comes when the body can not do so).

Where do you feel your stress?

_____

_____

_____

What emotions may be hidden there?

What feelings may need to be expressed?

Chapter 9: Stress-Inducing Self-Talk

Self-talk, or the tapes that we often play in our minds, can have both positive and negative effects. Some of the specific kinds of negative self-talk that can maintain stress include:

- Making mistakes is terrible.
- It is essential to be loved by everyone.
- I must always be competent.
- Every problem has a perfect solution.
- If others criticize me, I must have done something wrong.
- I can't change the way I think.
- I cannot show weakness or cry.
- Strong people do not ask for help.
- Everything is within my control.
- Other people should always see things the same way I do.

- ➢ People should do what I want because they love me.
- ➢ The world ought to be fair.

Negative self-talk can impact not only one's sense of well-being, but can also affect health and fertility.

What do you say to yourself?

_____

_____

_____

_____

_____

_____

_____

_____

_____

_____

_____

_____

Where did that self-talk come from?

_____

_____

_____

_____

_____

_____

_____

_____

_____

If you peel back the layers of time, whose voice fills your head? (We have discovered that while the voices sound like our own from first glance, if we track them back in time, they are often the negative or critical voices of our parents, coaches, or teachers)

_____

_____

_____

What is the self-talk that lessens your sense of self?

What is the self-talk that you hold on to that lowers your chance of conception?

_____

_____

_____

_____

_____

_____

_____

_____

What self-talk convinces your body to maintain disease and imbalance?

_____

_____

_____

Chapter 10: Stress-Reducing Self-Talk

Positive, or healthy self-talk can promote health, well-being and good self-esteem. Some examples of self-talk that can reduce stress are:

- ➢ This discomfort is time-limited. Nothing lasts forever.
- ➢ I have many options, not just one.
- ➢ I can make new choices whenever I want to.
- ➢ Breathe. With every breath, there is more relaxation.
- ➢ Relaxing helps my body work better.

What are the thoughts that help you relax?

Can you increase the number of frequency of those thoughts?

How can you create better balance?

Chapter 11: Nutrition: What are You Eating, or What's Eating You?

b. Current Diet

Make note of your current diet in the table below:

	Breakfast	Snack	Lunch	Snack	Dinner	Snack
Monday						
Tuesday						
Wednesday						

Thursday							
Friday							
Saturday							
Sunday							

How does your current diet support your fertility?

_____

_____

_____

_____

_____

_____

_____

What changes do you need to make?

_____

_____

_____

_____

_____

_____

_____

What changes will be challenging to incorporate?

_____

_____

_____

_____

_____

_____

_____

Use the below sheets to assess the food you eat and your exercise habits.

Name _____

Date: _____

Food Record

- This food record can help you and your nutritionist better understand how food affects your health
- Please write down everything you eat and drink from the time you wake up to the time you go to bed. Include meals, snacks, and drinks. If you eat or drink anything when you wake up, that should be added to the list.

Time	Type of food/Beverage	Amount

Name _____

Date: _____

Physical Activity History

- What type of activities do you do regularly and how much time each week do you spend doing then? Examples include walking, dancing, golf, tennis, biking aerobics, and swimming.

Activity	Times per Week	Minutes per Activity

- Do you like to do these activities alone or with others?

  _____

  _____

  _____

  _____

- Do you perform other physical activities of daily living, such as housework, gardening, or climbing stairs? If yes, list type and amount

  _____

  _____

  _____

  _____

  _____

  _____

- Are you interested in becoming more physically active?

_____ Yes, right now   _____ Yes, but I can't right now

_____ No, but I will think it over   _____ No, not now

_____ No, I'm not interested

If yes, what type of physical activity could you see yourself doing regularly?

_____

_____

_____

_____

_____

_____

If no, why not?

_____

_____

_____

_____

_____

Answer the following questions to see how well you fare with your diet:

- Do you eat 3 or more whole grain or enriched breads, cereals, rice, or pasta daily?

    ☐ Yes ☐ No

- Do you eat 2-3 pieces of fruit or drink 1-2 cups of juice daily?

    ☐ Yes ☐ No

- Do you eat 2-3 cups of raw or cooked vegetables daily?

    ☐ Yes ☐ No

- Do you drink 2 or more servings of skim milk and eat low fat or fat free dairy products daily?

    ☐ Yes ☐ No

- Do you not eat meat or trim fat from meat and take the skin off chicken and turkey?

    ☐ Yes ☐ No

- Do you not eat meat or eat small servings (size of a deck of cards) of meat poultry and fish?

  ☐ Yes   ☐ No

- Are most food and snacks that you eat made with no added fat (not fried) and no trans fats (partially hydrogenated vegetable oils)?

  ☐ Yes   ☐ No

- Do you add very little fat (butter, margarine, oil, or salad dressing) to your foods?

  ☐ Yes   ☐ No

- Do most dessert and snacks that you eat have no added sugar in them?

  ☐ Yes   ☐ No

- Is most of what you drink made without sugar or has no added sugar?

  ☐ Yes   ☐ No

- Do you rarely cook with salt or add it at the table?

  ☐ Yes   ☐ No

- Do you not drink alcohol or drink no more that 1-2 beers, 1-2 glasses of wine, or 1-2 mixed drinks daily?

  ☐ Yes   ☐ No

Please add up the number of statements answered yes to and compare that number with the scores listed below:

9-12   Great job! Eating "right" is one of the best things you can do to ensure good health. Daily exercise helps too.

5-8   You make some very good choices. Keep trying! Small changes in food habits can make a big difference.

0-4   Those first steps towards good eating are often the hardest to take. Making healthy choices gets easier everyday. You can do it?

The Food Pyramid

Since elementary school we have all been hearing about the food pyramid and how important it is to follow these guidelines. The Integrative Medicine department at the University of Michigan has created a NEW Food Pyramid for our modern times. This pyramid is more ideal the lifestyles we live and for our ability to conceive. Use this pyramid as your model for cooking and eating.

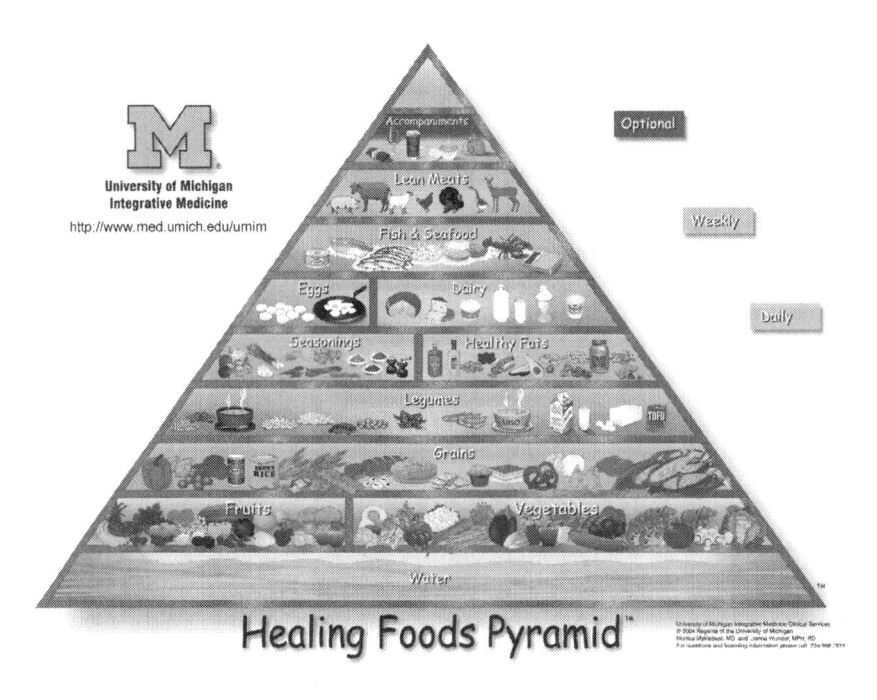

Below is a list of Fertility Super Foods that will nourish your body and improve your fertility. Take this list to the store with you and start adding these into your diet. Below are a few recipes that you use to start you down the right path.

Vegetables (3-5 servings daily)

Broccoli

Cabbage

Cauliflower

Spinach

Dark green leafy lettuce

Brussels sprouts

Collards

Bok choy

Swiss chard

Wheat grass

Yellow corn

Pumpkin

Carrots

Butternut squash

Yams

Sweet potatoes

Bell peppers

Artichoke hearts

Potatoes w/skin

Asparagus

Eggplant

Lentils

Black

Pinto

Kidney

Navy

Lima
Garbanzo
Green beans
Sugar snap peas
Green peas

Fruits (2-3 servings daily)
Blueberries
Raspberries
Strawberries
Blackberries
Boysenberries
Cranberries
Cherries
Dried prunes
Plums
Purple grapes
Pomegranate
Oranges
Lemons
Limes
Grapefruit
Tangerines
Watermelon
Tomatoes
Papaya

Peaches

Cantaloupe

Mango

Apples

Apricots

Whole Grains (6-11 servings)

Oatmeal

Oat Bran

Wheat germ

Brown rice

Wild rice

Barley

Whole wheat

Buckwheat

Rye

Millet

Bulgur wheat

Amaranth

Quinoa

Triticale

Kamut

Spelt

Dairy (2-3 servings daily)

Organic Yogurt

Kefir

Soy
Tempeh
Miso

Protein (2-3 servings daily)
Skinless turkey breast
Skinless chicken breast
Wild Salmon
Alaskan halibut
Albacore tuna
Omega-3 enriched eggs

Fats (sparingly)
Avocados
Extra-virgin olive oil
Coconut Oil
Walnuts
Almonds
Peanuts
Pecans
Cashews
Pistachios
Brazil nuts

Seeds

Sesame seeds

Sunflower seeds

Pumpkin seeds

Flaxseed

Tea

Green tea

White tea

Black tea

Oolong tea

Seasonings

Red/white onion

Garlic

Ginger

Cinnamon

Parsley/Rosemary

Oregano/ Basil

Chives/Cilantro

Dill/Mint

Citrus zest

Sometimes, it's difficult knowing how to make great-tasting dishes with the ingredients of a new diet. Below are some tried and true recipes for your health and fertility!

Recipes

Power Pilaf
Prep: 10 min, Cook: 10 min.

For 4 servings:
- 2 tsp. olive oil
- 1-1/4 medium carrots\raw, thinly sliced
- 1-1/3 cups broccoli florets raw
- 1 clove garlic, minced
- 1/2 cup spicy vegetable juice
- 1 Tbs. plus 1 tsp. Worcestershire sauce, regular or low-sodium
- 1-1/4 tsp. dried thyme leaves
- 1/4 tsp. salt
- 1/8 tsp. ground black pepper
- 4 cups cooked rice
- 10 ounces canned black beans, drained and rinsed
- 10 ounces canned kidney beans, drained and rinsed

Heat oil in large skillet over medium-high heat until hot. Add carrots, broccoli, onion, and garlic. Cook 4-5 minutes, or until vegetables are crisp-tender. Add vegetable juice, Worcestershire sauce, thyme, salt, and pepper. Stir in rice, black beans, and kidney beans. Cook 2-3 minutes more until thoroughly heated. You can serve this dish by itself or with grilled chicken breasts or pork chops. Courtesy American Dry Bean Board.

Per serving: calories 411, fat 3.6g, 8% calories from fat, cholesterol 0mg, protein 14.2g, carbohydrates 80.9g, fiber 9.9g, sugar 7g, sodium 429mg, diet points 7.0

Serving Nutritional Information For 4 Servings of: Power Pilaf.				
Nutrients		**Exchanges**		
Calories	411	Diet Points		7.0
Protein	14.2g	Milk Exchanges		0
Carbohydrates	80.9g	Vegetable Exchanges		1
Dietary Fiber	9.9g	Fruit Exchanges		0
Sugar	7.0g	Bread Exchanges		4.5
Fat Total	3.6g	Other Carbohydrates/Sugar Exchanges		0
Saturated Fat	2.8g	Lean Meat Exchanges		0
Mono-unsaturated Fat	3.9g	Very Lean Meat/Protein Exchanges		0.5
Poly-unsaturated Fat	2.2g	Fat Exchanges		0.5
% Calories from Fat	7.9%	The color green indicates that the recipes provide a beneficial source of a nutrient, as defined by the US RDA, prorated for a 2000-calorie diet.		
Cholesterol	0mg	^		
Sodium	429mg	^		
Vitamins	% RDA	**Minerals**		% RDA
Vitamin A	707 IU	14%	Calcium	100mg	10%
Thiamin (B1)	1.02mg	68%	Copper	1.81mg	91%
Riboflavin (B2)	1.09mg	64%	Iron	5.8mg	32%
Niacin (B3)	4.2mg	21%	Magnesium	84mg	21%
Vitamin B6	2.73mg	136%	Manganese	1.36mg	55%
Vitamin B12	0.00mcg	0%	Phosphorus	267mg	27%
Vitamin C	36.5mg	61%	Potassium	726mg	21%
Vitamin E	3.2 IU	11%	Selenium	26.1mcg	37%
Folate	111mcg	56%	Sodium	429mg	18%
Pantothentic Acid	1.21mg	12%	Zinc	1.9mg	13%

Black Bean, Corn and Tomato Salad
Prep: 5 min, Marinate: 15 min, Cook: 5 min.

For 4 servings:
- 1/4 cup fresh lemon juice
- 3 Tbs. olive oil
- 2 cups corn kernels, thawed if frozen
- 2 lbs. canned black beans, rinsed and drained
- 4 plum tomatoes, seeded and chopped
- 2 scallions, minced
- 1/4 cup fresh parsley, minced
- 1/8 tsp. cayenne
- 8 lettuce leaves

Combine lemon juice, oil and salt to taste in a jar with a tight fitting lid. Shake vigorously. Place corn in a steamer basket over boiling water. Cover pan and steam 3-4 minutes, or until just cooked. Drain and combine with remaining ingredients, except lettuce. Season with salt and pepper to taste. **Set aside** 15 minutes, stirring occasionally. Serve salad over lettuce leaves.

Per serving: calories 404, fat 12.2g, 26% calories from fat, cholesterol 0mg, protein 17.7g, carbohydrates 61.9g, fiber 19.7g, sugar 15.4g, sodium 409mg, diet points 5.7.

Per Serving Nutritional Information For 4 Servings of: Black Bean, Corn and Tomato Salad.				
Nutrients			**Exchanges**	
Calories		404	Diet Points	5.7
Protein		17.7g	Milk Exchanges	0
Carbohydrates		61.9g	Vegetable Exchanges	1.5
Dietary Fiber		19.7g	Fruit Exchanges	0
Sugar		15.4g	Bread Exchanges	3.5
Fat Total		12.2g	Other Carbohydrates/Sugar Exchanges	0
Saturated Fat		3.8g	Lean Meat Exchanges	0
Mono-unsaturated Fat		9.2g	Very Lean Meat/Protein Exchanges	0
Poly-unsaturated Fat		1.9g	Fat Exchanges	2
% Calories from Fat		25.6%	The color green indicates that the recipes provide a beneficial source of a nutrient, as defined by the US RDA, prorated for a 2000-calorie diet.	
Cholesterol		0mg		
Sodium		409mg		
Vitamins		% RDA	**Minerals**	% RDA
Vitamin A	137 IU	3%	Calcium	115mg	11%
Thiamin (B1)	1.66mg	110%	Copper	2.03mg	102%
Riboflavin (B2)	1.67mg	98%	Iron	6.5mg	36%
Niacin (B3)	3.4mg	17%	Magnesium	119mg	30%
Vitamin B6	2.80mg	140%	Manganese	1.03mg	41%
Vitamin B12	0.00mcg	0%	Phosphorus	344mg	34%
Vitamin C	62.6mg	104%	Potassium	1276mg	36%
Vitamin E	4.0 IU	13%	Selenium	1.3mcg	2%
Folate	235mcg	117%	Sodium	409mg	17%
Pantothentic Acid	1.36mg	14%	Zinc	2.9mg	19%

Quick Chicken Tostadas
Prep: 10 min, Cook: 5 min.

For 4 servings:
- 4 large flour tortillas
- 1/2 cup canned refried beans
- 1/2 cup salsa
- 3/4 lb. roasted chicken meat, chopped
- 4 green onions, chopped
- 1 cup fat-free cheddar cheese
- 1/2 cup nonfat sour cream
- 2 cups lettuce, shredded
- 2 medium tomatoes, chopped

Turn on broiler. Arrange tortillas on a cookie sheet. Spread refried beans over tortillas. Add salsa, and then layer with chicken, onions, and cheese. Place cookie sheet under broiler 1-2 minutes or until the cheese melts and the tortillas are crisp. Serve topped with sour cream, lettuce and tomatoes.

Per serving: calories 553, fat 9.1g, 15% calories from fat, cholesterol 80mg, protein 48.9g, carbohydrates 67.3g, fiber 7.5g, sugar 13.8g, sodium 874mg, diet points 10.8.

Per Serving Nutritional Information For 4 Servings of: Quick Chicken Tostadas.			
Nutrients		**Exchanges**	
Calories	553	Diet Points	10.8
Protein	48.9g	Milk Exchanges	0
Carbohydrates	67.3g	Vegetable Exchanges	3
Dietary Fiber	7.5g	Fruit Exchanges	0
Sugar	13.8g	Bread Exchanges	3
Fat Total	9.1g	Other Carbohydrates/Sugar Exchanges	0
Saturated Fat	2.6g	Lean Meat Exchanges	0
Mono-unsaturated Fat	4.2g	Very Lean Meat/Protein Exchanges	4.5
Poly-unsaturated Fat	3.8g	Fat Exchanges	1
% Calories from Fat	14.9%	The color green indicates that the recipes provide a beneficial source of a nutrient, as defined by the US RDA, prorated for a 2000-calorie diet.	
Cholesterol	80mg		
Sodium	874mg		
Vitamins || % RDA	**Minerals** || % RDA

Vitamins		% RDA	Minerals		% RDA
Vitamin A	278 IU	6%	Calcium	443mg	44%
Thiamin (B1)	2.23mg	149%	Copper	2.10mg	105%
Riboflavin (B2)	1.99mg	117%	Iron	4.5mg	25%
Niacin (B3)	15.1mg	75%	Magnesium	87mg	22%
Vitamin B6	1.94mg	97%	Manganese	0.83mg	33%
Vitamin B12	0.65mcg	32%	Phosphorus	568mg	57%
Vitamin C	34.4mg	57%	Potassium	935mg	27%
Vitamin E	2.9 IU	10%	Selenium	43.2mcg	62%
Folate	72mcg	36%	Sodium	874mg	36%
Pantothentic Acid	1.96mg	20%	Zinc	3.8mg	25%

Baked Mahi-Mahi

Prep: 5 min, Marinate: 10 min, Cook: 20 min.

For 4 servings:
- 1 mahi-mahi or red snapper fillet, about 1-1/2 lbs. each
- 1/4 cup orange juice
- 2 Tbs. lemon juice
- 3/4 tsp. cornstarch
- 1-1/2 Tbs. water
- 1 Tbs. orange marmalade
- 1 Tbs. lemon zest

Preheat oven to 400°F. Spray a non-reactive baking dish with cooking spray. Arrange fish fillets in dish. Drizzle with orange and lemon juice. Season with salt and pepper to taste. **Set aside** 10-15 minutes, turning once to marinate. **Bake** fish 12-15 minutes or until fish flakes easily. Transfer fish fillets to a platter, cover and keep warm. Pour fish juice from baking dish into a heavy saucepan. Dissolve cornstarch in water. Stir into fish juice. Add marmalade and lemon zest. Stir over medium high heat 3-4 minutes or until sauce thickens. Serve sauce over fish.

Per serving: calories 78, fat 0.8g, 9% calories from fat, cholesterol 20mg, protein 11.3g, carbohydrates 6.3g, fiber 0.2g, sugar 5.1g, sodium 38mg, diet points 2.1.

Per Serving Nutritional Information For 4 Servings of: Baked Mahi-Mahi.			
Nutrients		Exchanges	
Calories	78	Diet Points	2.1
Protein	11.3g	Milk Exchanges	0
Carbohydrates	6.3g	Vegetable Exchanges	0
Dietary Fiber	0.2g	Fruit Exchanges	0
Sugar	5.1g	Bread Exchanges	0
Fat Total	0.8g	Other Carbohydrates/Sugar Exchanges	0
Saturated Fat	0.2g	Lean Meat Exchanges	0
Mono-unsaturated Fat	0.2g	Very Lean Meat/Protein Exchanges	1.5
Poly-unsaturated Fat	0.3g	Fat Exchanges	0
% Calories from Fat	8.9%	The color green indicates that the recipes provide a beneficial source of a nutrient, as defined by the US RDA, prorated for a 2000-calorie diet.	
Cholesterol	20mg		
Sodium	38mg		
Vitamins	% RDA	Minerals	% RDA
Vitamin A	20 IU	0%	Calcium	24mg	2%
Thiamin (B1)	0.45mg	30%	Copper	0.34mg	17%
Riboflavin (B2)	0.26mg	15%	Iron	0.2mg	1%
Niacin (B3)	0.3mg	1%	Magnesium	20mg	5%
Vitamin B6	0.33mg	16%	Manganese	0.17mg	7%
Vitamin B12	1.64mcg	82%	Phosphorus	112mg	11%
Vitamin C	14.3mg	24%	Potassium	272mg	8%
Vitamin E	0.4 IU	1%	Selenium	21.0mcg	30%
Folate	10mcg	5%	Sodium	38mg	2%
Pantothentic Acid	0.46mg	5%	Zinc	0.4mg	2%

Black Bean and Pumpkin Soup
Prep: 10 min, Cook: 15 min.

- 3/4 ancho pepper
- 3/4 tsp. cumin seeds
- 10 ounces canned black beans, rinsed, drained
- 2/3 cup onions\raw, chopped
- 2 cloves garlic, peeled
- 1-1/3 cups vegetable broth, or fat-free reduced-sodium chicken broth
- 2/3 cup water
- 10 ounces pumpkin
- 1/8 tsp. cilantro, finely chopped

Heat ancho pepper in dry skillet over medium heat until softened; remove chili and discard veins and seeds. Add cumin seeds to skillet; **cook** until toasted, about 30 seconds (watch carefully and do not burn). Process ancho chili, cumin seeds, black beans, onions, garlic, broth, and water at high speed in blender until smooth.

Transfer bean mixture to saucepan; stir in pumpkin and heat to boiling. Reduce heat and simmer, covered, 5 minutes; season to taste with salt and pepper. Serve in bowls; sprinkle with cilantro. This soup can also be served chilled.

You can make this soup 2-3 days in advance; it can be frozen up to 2 months.

Courtesy American Dry Bean Board.
Dietary Exchanges: Milk: 0.0, Vegetable: 0.7, Fruit: 0.0, Bread: 1.0, Lean meat: 0.0, Fat: 0.0, Sugar: 0.0, Very lean meat protein: 0.0

Per serving: calories 103, fat 1.1g, 9% calories from fat, cholesterol 0mg, protein 5.7g, carbohydrates 20.2g, fiber 6.5g, sugar 7.5g, sodium 331mg,.

Per Serving Nutritional Information For 4 Servings of: Black Bean and Pumpkin Soup.

Nutrients		Exchanges	
Calories	103	Diet Points	1.3
Protein	5.7g	Milk Exchanges	0
Carbohydrates	20.2g	Vegetable Exchanges	1
Dietary Fiber	6.5g	Fruit Exchanges	0
Sugar	7.5g	Bread Exchanges	1
Fat Total	1.1g	Other Carbohydrates/Sugar Exchanges	0
Saturated Fat	0.9g	Lean Meat Exchanges	0
Mono-unsaturated Fat	0.4g	Very Lean Meat/Protein Exchanges	0
Poly-unsaturated Fat	0.7g	Fat Exchanges	0
% Calories from Fat	8.5%	The color green indicates that the recipes provide a beneficial source of a nutrient, as defined by the US RDA, prorated for a 2000 calorie diet.	
Cholesterol	0mg		
Sodium	331mg		

Vitamins		% RDA	Minerals		% RDA
Vitamin A	959 IU	19%	Calcium	53mg	5%
Thiamin (B1)	0.58mg	39%	Copper	1.21mg	61%
Riboflavin (B2)	0.84mg	49%	Iron	2.3mg	13%
Niacin (B3)	1.0mg	5%	Magnesium	40mg	10%
Vitamin B6	0.80mg	40%	Manganese	0.95mg	38%
Vitamin B12	0.00mcg	0%	Phosphorus	119mg	12%
Vitamin C	46.1mg	77%	Potassium	501mg	14%
Vitamin E	1.6 IU	5%	Selenium	0.7mcg	1%
Folate	58mcg	29%	Sodium	331mg	14%
Pantothentic Acid	0.41mg	4%	Zinc	0.8mg	5%

Santa Fe Bean Mashers
Prep: 25 min, Cook: 35 min.

- 1 lb. canned navy beans, rinsed and drained
- 2 medium potatoes, peeled and cut into small cubes
- 3/4 cup nonfat milk
- 2 Tbs. cooking oil
- 1 medium poblano chilli, chopped
- 1 tsp. garlic, minced
- 1/4 lb. reduced fat sharp cheddar cheese
- 1/8 tsp. salt (optional)
- 1/8 tsp. black pepper (optional)

Heat beans, potatoes and milk to boiling in medium saucepan. Reduce heat and **simmer**, covered, 10 minutes. Uncover and simmer until potatoes are tender and milk is almost absorbed, about 10 minutes longer, stirring frequently to prevent sticking.

Spray small skillet with cooking spray; heat over medium heat until hot. Sauté poblano chile and garlic until tender, 8-10 minutes.

Beat bean mixture with electric mixer at high speed until smooth; mix in poblano chile mixture. Return mixture to saucepan and heat over medium heat until hot. Remove from heat and stir in cheese. Season to taste with salt and pepper.

Courtesy American Dry Bean Board.

Dietary Exchanges: Milk: 0.2, Vegetable: 0.2, Fruit: 0.0, Bread: 3.8, Lean meat: 0.0, Fat: 1.3, Sugar: 0.0, Very lean meat protein: 0.0

Per serving: calories 395, fat 7.4g, 17% calories from fat, cholesterol 5mg, protein 18.9g, carbohydrates 64.2g, fiber 8.6g, sugar 12.7g, sodium 473mg.

Per Serving Nutritional Information For 4 Servings of: Santa Fe Bean Mashers.

Nutrients		Exchanges	
Calories	395	Diet Points	7.3
Protein	18.9g	Milk Exchanges	0
Carbohydrates	64.2g	Vegetable Exchanges	0
Dietary Fiber	8.6g	Fruit Exchanges	0
Sugar	12.7g	Bread Exchanges	4
Fat Total	7.4g	Other Carbohydrates/Sugar Exchanges	0
Saturated Fat	1.7g	Lean Meat Exchanges	0
Mono-unsaturated Fat	4.8g	Very Lean Meat/Protein Exchanges	0
Poly-unsaturated Fat	3.0g	Fat Exchanges	1.5
% Calories from Fat	16.6%	The color green indicates that the recipes provide a beneficial source of a nutrient, as defined by the US RDA, prorated for a 2000 calorie diet.	
Cholesterol	5mg		
Sodium	473mg		
Vitamins	**% RDA**	**Minerals**	**% RDA**
Vitamin A	165 IU	3%	Calcium	379mg	38%
Thiamin (B1)	1.49mg	99%	Copper	0.72mg	36%
Riboflavin (B2)	2.01mg	118%	Iron	5.4mg	30%
Niacin (B3)	2.7mg	13%	Magnesium	100mg	25%
Vitamin B6	1.51mg	75%	Manganese	1.00mg	40%
Vitamin B12	0.17mcg	9%	Phosphorus	1292mg	129%
Vitamin C	44.1mg	73%	Potassium	1235mg	35%
Vitamin E	3.8 IU	13%	Selenium	2.7mcg	4%
Folate	93mcg	46%	Sodium	473mg	20%
Pantothentic Acid	1.12mg	11%	Zinc	1.9mg	13%

Skillet Chili
Prep: 5 min, Cook: 15 min.

- 1 Tbs. olive oil
- 2 onions\cooked, chopped
- 2 green bell peppers\cooked, seeded and chopped
- 2 Tbs. chili powder
- 3-3/4 cups Mexican style stewed tomatoes
- 2 lbs. canned pinto beans, drained
- 1 cup water
- 3 cups fat-free Monterey Jack cheese, grated, with jalapeño peppers, if desired

Prepare broiler. Heat oil in a heavy ovenproof skillet over medium high heat. Sauté onion and bell pepper about 4 minutes, stirring occasionally, until softened and lightly browned. Add chili powder and cook another minute. Stir in tomatoes, beans and water. Bring to a boil over high heat. Reduce heat to medium and **simmer** 8-10 minutes, until thickened. Sprinkle with cheese and broil 4 inches from heat source about 1 minute, or until cheese is melted.

Dietary Exchanges: Milk: 0.0, Vegetable: 4.6, Fruit: 0.0, Bread: 2.3, Lean meat: 0.0, Fat: 0.7, Sugar: 0.0, Very lean meat protein: 3.3

Per serving: calories 456, fat 6.4g, 12% calories from fat, cholesterol 8mg, protein 41.5g, carbohydrates 60.2g, fiber 15.5g, sugar 18.8g, sodium 1274mg.

Per Serving Nutritional Information For 4 Servings of: Skillet Chili.

Nutrients		Exchanges	
Calories	456	Diet Points	7.1
Protein	41.5g	Milk Exchanges	0
Carbohydrates	60.2g	Vegetable Exchanges	4.5
Dietary Fiber	15.5g	Fruit Exchanges	0
Sugar	18.8g	Bread Exchanges	2.5
Fat Total	6.4g	Other Carbohydrates/Sugar Exchanges	0
Saturated Fat	1.7g	Lean Meat Exchanges	0
Mono-unsaturated Fat	3.7g	Very Lean Meat/Protein Exchanges	3.5
Poly-unsaturated Fat	3.1g	Fat Exchanges	0.5
% Calories from Fat	12.3%	The color green indicates that the recipes provide a beneficial source of a nutrient, as defined by the US RDA, prorated for a 2000 calorie diet.	
Cholesterol	8mg		
Sodium	1274mg		
Vitamins		**% RDA**	**Minerals**		**% RDA**

Vitamins		% RDA	Minerals		% RDA
Vitamin A	578 IU	12%	Calcium	1525mg	153%
Thiamin (B1)	1.80mg	120%	Copper	1.69mg	84%
Riboflavin (B2)	2.44mg	144%	Iron	5.5mg	31%
Niacin (B3)	2.9mg	15%	Magnesium	107mg	27%
Vitamin B6	3.96mg	198%	Manganese	1.11mg	44%
Vitamin B12	0.00mcg	0%	Phosphorus	296mg	30%
Vitamin C	68.6mg	114%	Potassium	1309mg	37%
Vitamin E	5.5 IU	18%	Selenium	19.4mcg	28%
Folate	175mcg	88%	Sodium	1274mg	53%
Pantothentic Acid	1.07mg	11%	Zinc	2.4mg	16%

Making a plan of Action:

Now use this sheet to set a plane of action. How do you want to change things? What do you want to add your diet and lifestyle to make positive changes toward a healthier life and to increase your ability to conceive?

Nutrition & Exercise Assessment

Name _____

Date _____

Ht: Current Wt: BMI:

Wt range past 5 yrs: Goal Wt:

Current	**Goal/Plan**
Fruits/Veggies	
Whole Grains	
Dairy/Calcium Rich	
Lean Proteins	
Fats	
Fluids	
Supplements	
Eating Out	

Current	**Exercise Goal/Plan**
Cardio	
Strength Training	
Flexibility	

Sample Meal Plan

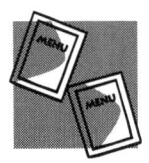

Breakfast	
Snack	
Lunch	
Snack	
Dinner	
Snack	

Chapter 12: Relaxation Exercises

Most of the relaxation exercises included in this workbook are also available in audio version on the Conception CD.

c. Mindful Meditation

Meditation involves the practice of focusing on your internal state and learning to quiet the mind, body and spirit, *at will*, with the help of the breath. Experiment with the Meditation Exercise below:

➢ Stretch out on the ground or find a comfortable position on your chair, couch or bed.

➢ Turn the lights down if possible and make sure that you have enough space around you.

➢ Close your eyes if you are willing, though this is not necessary.

- Take a deep breath from the belly (you can practice this with your eyes open so that you can watch your belly distend with air as you breathe deeply).
- Focus on the experience of the breath and your body's reaction to each breath.
- Repeat the deep breath, observing how tense muscles relax as oxygen flows there with each breath.
- Breathe normally, continuing to focus on each inhale and each exhale.
- For a deeper experience, count to four as you inhale, and count to four as you exhale.
- Finish with a deep breath, then open your eyes.

What was it like to focus only on your breath for a few minutes?

_____

_____

_____

_____

_____

What response did you notice, if any, in your body?

_____

_____

_____

_____

_____

_____

_____

_____

_____

d. Autogenic Training

Autogenic Training combines a set of "suggestions" for the body with the practice of basic meditation. Suggestions are aimed at enabling the body to feel heavy and warm- much like you feel just before you drift off to sleep. Try the exercise below to induce the Relaxation Response!

➢ Sit in a balanced position in your chair. Move your feet around until the feet are comfortably placed on the floor. Lift your hands in the air, then let them fall to your lap.

- Close your eyes if you are willing to do so.
- Visualize your head being held up by strings. Now visualize the strings being cut, allowing your head to fall forward until a comfortable position is reached.
- Focus on each body part one at a time, and to repeat silently the following statements three times each:
    - My right hand is heavy and warm.
    - My left hand is heavy and warm.
    - My right foot is heavy and warm.
    - My left foot is heavy and warm.
    - My hands and feet are heavy and warm.
    - My abdomen is warm.
    - My breathing is deep, relaxed and comfortable.
    - My heartbeat is calm and regular.
    - My shoulders are heavy and warm.
    - My jaw is heavy and relaxed.
    - My forehead is cool and relaxed.
    - My mind is calm and serene.
    - A relaxing warmth flows throughout my entire body.
    - My whole body feels comfortable and relaxed.
    - I am at peace.

➢ Take a moment and let your eyes open slowly.

What was this process like?

_____

_____

_____

_____

_____

_____

_____

How did it differ from the simple meditation?

_____

_____

_____

How was it positive? Negative?

e. Progressive Relaxation

If it's hard for you to simply *command* your body to relax, you may do better with *Progressive Relaxation*. During Progressive Relaxation, you first contract your muscles, then release, or relax, the muscle group. If you sometimes have trouble with spontaneous relaxation, give the exercise below a try.

➢ *Stretch out on the floor, in a chair, on the couch or on your bed. Get as comfortable as possible, and close your eyes if you are able.*

➢ *Breathe deeply and bring your focus to your face.*

➢ *Squinch or crumple your face as tightly as possible and hold the pose for 3 seconds (count to 3 silently). At the end of the 3-count, breathe deeply and relax your face.*

➢ *Contract your shoulders as tightly as possible (touch your ears to your shoulders) and hold the pose for 3 seconds (count to 3 silently). At the end of the 3-count, breathe deeply and relax your shoulders.*

➢ *Contract your arms as tightly as possible (pull your fists into your shoulders, flexing the biceps) and hold the pose for 3 seconds (count to 3 silently). At the end of the 3-count, breathe deeply and relax your arms by stretching them out straight in front of you.*

➢ *Contract your buttocks as tightly as possible (squeeze the gluts as if they were trying to hold a penny between your cheeks!) and hold the pose for 3 seconds (count to 3 silently). At the end of the 3-count, breathe deeply and relax your buttocks.*

➢ *Contract your legs as tightly as possible (straighten your legs out in front of you, flexing the feet back towards you) and hold the pose for 3 seconds (count to 3 silently). At the end of the 3-count, breathe deeply and relax your legs.*

➢ *Contract your feet as tightly as possible (curl your toes down, as if to make a ball with the feet) and hold the pose for 3 seconds (count to 3 silently). At the end of* the 3-count, breathe deeply and relax your feet. If you get a foot cramp, simply stretch your feet back towards the body and breathe deeply.

> *Finally, take a deep belly breath and exhale with vigor. Follow this with a deep inhale, and a slow exhale.*

How did this form of relaxation compare to the others?

_____

_____

_____

_____

_____

Was it easier to relax by engaging the muscles to do so?

_____

_____

_____

_____

f. Passive Progressive Relaxation

Through Passive Progressive Relaxation, you can sequentially relax parts of the body by sending soothing messages one at a time, rather than requiring the muscle to work so that it will relax. Passive Progressive Relaxation combines a series of breaths and images to help you relax. Sometimes you'll breathe deeply, all the way into your belly, and sometimes you'll just use a regular breath.

Give it a try!

➢ Find a comfortable posture, either seated, reclined, lying on the floor or bed.

➢ Take a deep breath. As you inhale, bring your attention to the top of your head. As you exhale, imagine all the muscles in your scalp letting go.

➢ Breathe deeply again and focus on your scalp. As you exhale, let go of all the muscles in your scalp.

➢ Breathe normally.

➢ When you are ready, breathe deeply again and as you inhale, bring your attention to the muscles in your face. As you exhale, let go of all the muscles in your face.

➢ Imagine that you are standing under a wonderfully soothing waterfall, cool, but not cold, and warm, but not hot. Feel the water gently massaging your scalp and face, rinsing all the stress away so that it drips off your fingertips.

➢ Take another deep breath and focus on any tension in your shoulders. As you exhale, let go of all the muscles in your shoulders. Imagine the water washing over your head, face and shoulders, just rinsing away the stress until it drips off your fingertips. Breathe normally as the stress washes away.

➢ When you are ready, breathe deeply in. As you inhale, focus on your back. As you exhale, imagine the waterfall washing away any stress or tension remaining there. Let your breath carry away any remnants of stress.

➢ Breathe deeply and focus on any tension in your arms. As you exhale, let go of all the muscles in your arms. Imagine the water washing over your head, face, shoulders, back and arms and rinsing away the stress until it drips off your fingertips. Breathe normally as the stress washes away.

➢ Take another deep breath directly into your torso and pelvis. As you exhale, let go of all the muscles in those areas.

➢ Breathe deeply again and focus on any tension in your legs. As you exhale, let go of all the muscles in your legs, knees, and shins. Imagine the water washing over your head, face, shoulders, back, arms, torso, pelvis, legs, knees and shins and rinsing away the stress until it drips off your toes. Breathe normally as the stress washes away.

➢ Take another deep breath. As you inhale, focus on your ankles, heels and feet. As you exhale, let go of any tension there.

➢ Breathe deeply one last time and focus on tension remaining in your head and face. As you exhale, imagine letting go of any stress there. Imagine the waterfall washing over your head, face, shoulders, back, arms, torso, pelvis, legs, knees and shins, ankles, heels and feet and rinsing away the stress until it drips off your fingers and toes.

➢ Breathe normally as you watch and feel the stress wash away.

➢ When you are ready, take one last breath and allow your eyes to open.

How was that for you?

_____

_____

_____

_____

_____

How did this form of relaxation exercise differ from the others?

Do you feel any different using this strategy?

Which of the relaxation techniques did you most prefer?

Which was the most effective for you?

Chapter 13: Yoga : Postures for Optimal Health & Fertility

Yoga Postures for Fertility

Some of the Yoga poses which may improve fertility include:

- **Pranayama (Abdominal Breathing)**
  This pose is designed to calm the nervous system, create feelings of connectedness between mind and body, and trigger the relaxation response.

    o Come to a comfortable seated position, pulling the flesh back on your rear so you can sit directly on your sitting bones (to help lengthen your spine, sit on the edge of a folded blanket.)

- Invite the lower half of your body from your pelvis down to release into the ground, relaxing your knees, hips, and ankles.
- Lengthen up from the crown of your head, extending your spine into a tall and straight position.
- Allow your shoulders to relax down away from your ears and your hands to rest on your knees.
- Close your mouth and breathe through your nose. As you inhale, take your breath all the way down into your belly.
- Allow your belly to be soft so it expands with the breath. Pause for a moment and then slowly exhale. Pause again briefly after the exhale and continue with this slow deep breathing. Allow the breath to travel into your sides and back as well as if you had a band wrapped around your belly and you were trying to expand the band in all directions. Work on keeping your breath smooth and relaxed.
- Now as you inhale, imagine your breath as white light filled with healing energy that is being sent to every part of your body. As you exhale, imagine all of your worries and stresses draining from your body with the breath.

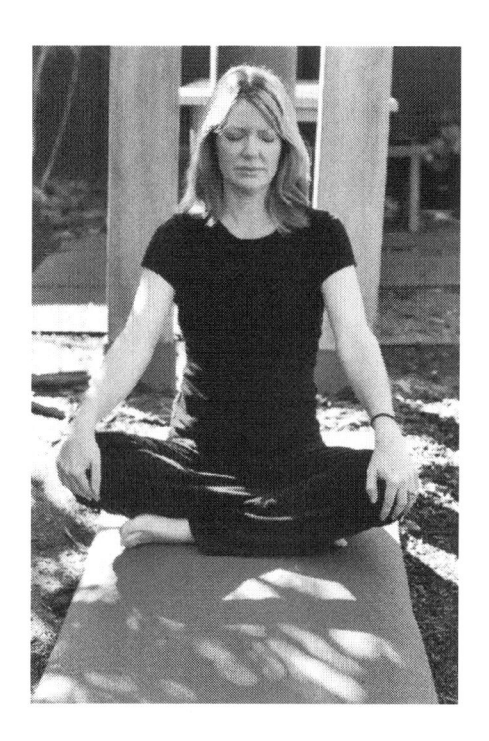

- **Vajrasana (Thunderbolt Pose)**

    This pose is designed to strengthen the pelvic muscles.

    - o Kneel on the floor with your knees all the way together and your big toes touching.
    - o Allow your heels to separate slightly.
    - o Sit back onto the soles of your feet with the heels touching the sides of your hips.
    - o Place your hands on your knees, palms down.

- o Lengthen up through your back and pull your naval in towards your spine to reduce arching of the low back.
- o Relax your arms and allow your breath to flow through your abdomen.

Modification: If you feel pain in the thighs, separate the knees slightly. Place a folded blanket between your rear and the heels for added comfort.

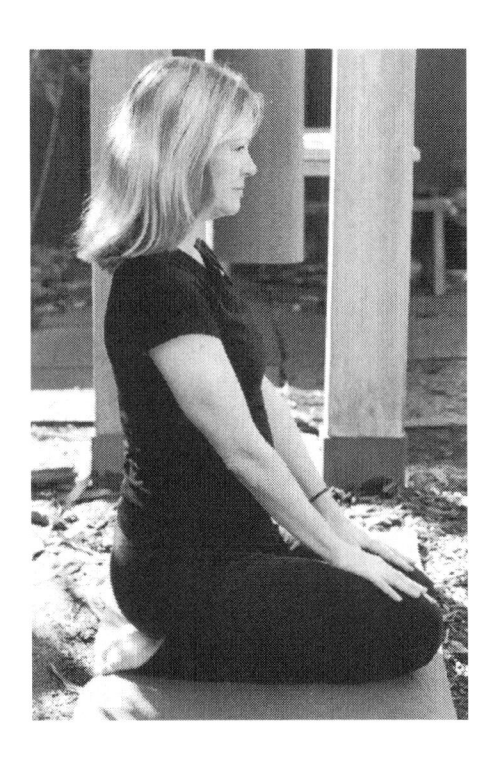

- **Balasana (Child's Pose)**

This pose promotes calm for the nervous system, massages the abdominal organs, kidneys and adrenal glands, and heals, rejuvenates and relaxes the entire body and mind.

- Start in a hands and knees position with the big toes touching.
- Sit your rear back to your heels and extend your torso out with your forehead resting on the ground.
- Keep the arms relaxed alongside your body with the palms facing up.
- Allow your breath to expand into your sides and back.
- Soften and release all your muscles and bones and allow the circulation to penetrate every organ and cell in your body.
- Release your abdominal muscles and breathe into your pelvic area.

Modification: If the forward fold feels too intense, fold a blanket in front of you and rest your forehead on it.

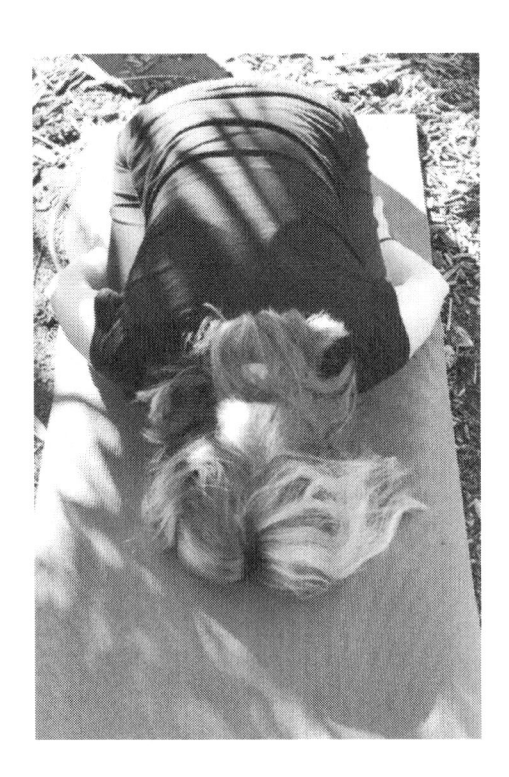

- **Malasana (Squat Pose)**

    This pose is designed to open the hips and groin area, provides a massage for the abdominal and reproductive organs, and provides relief from menstrual cramps.

    - Stand with the feet a little wider than hips distance apart with the toes turned slightly outward.
    - Bend your knees and lower all the way to the ground with the heels to the floor.
    - Bring the elbows between the knees with the palms pressing together at the heart center.

- As the hands press together, use the elbows to help open the knees a little wider.
- With each inhalation, draw breath into the core of your being and release any tension in the abdomen or pelvic floor.
- Maintain a relaxed, steady breathing pattern.

Modification: If your heels do not reach the floor, place a folded blanket underneath each of the heels for support, allowing your body to relax into the pose.

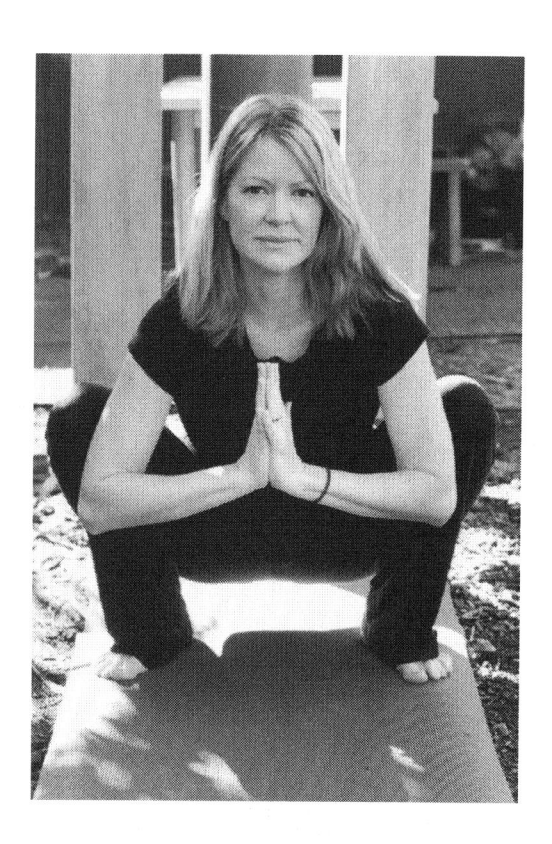

- **Paschimottanasana (Seated Forward Bend)**

    This pose massages the abdominal organs and reproductive system, and can calm anxiety.

    - Sit on the ground with the legs extend in front of you so that the ankle bones are touching.
    - As you inhale, lengthen the spine and lift the arms up and over the head, as you exhale, fold forward leading with your heart.
    - Allow your hands to rest wherever they reach (floor, legs, or feet).

- o As you inhale, work on lengthening the spine and feeling the crown of the head reaching towards the toes.
- o As you exhale, allow the body to relax into the fold, releasing the head and neck.

Modification: To help lengthen the spine and become more comfortable in the pose, place a folded blanket underneath the sitting bones, allowing your pelvis to tilt forward.

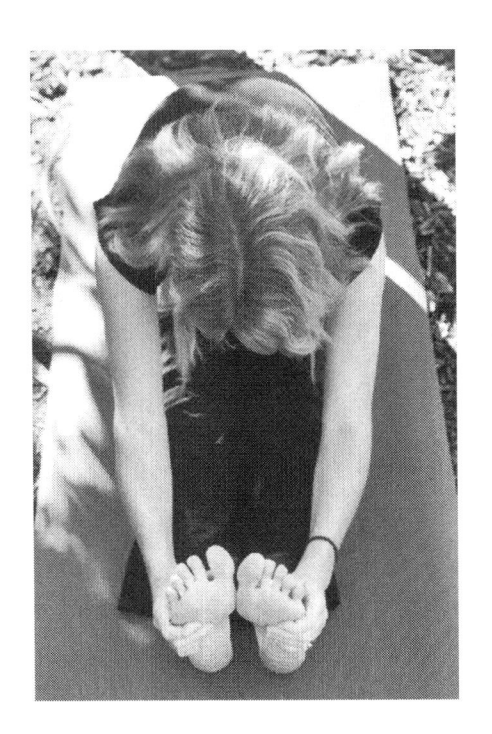

- **Janu Sirsasana (Head to Knee Pose)**

This pose tones the reproductive organs and their supporting muscles, as well as brings a sense of peace if you are feeling agitated.

- Sit on the floor with both legs extended in front of you.
- Bend your right knee to a 45 degree angle to the left leg.
- Place the sole of the right foot high on the inner thigh of the left leg.
- Pull the heel close into the groin.
- Use the right hand to take a hold of the outside of the left leg or foot.
- Inhale to lengthen the spine and as you exhale use the hand to help twist the torso so it is situated directly over the left leg.
- Work on bringing the naval directly over the middle of the left thigh.
- Use your inhale to extend the torso out over the leg and relax into the pose on the exhale.
- Remember to perform the pose on the other side as well.

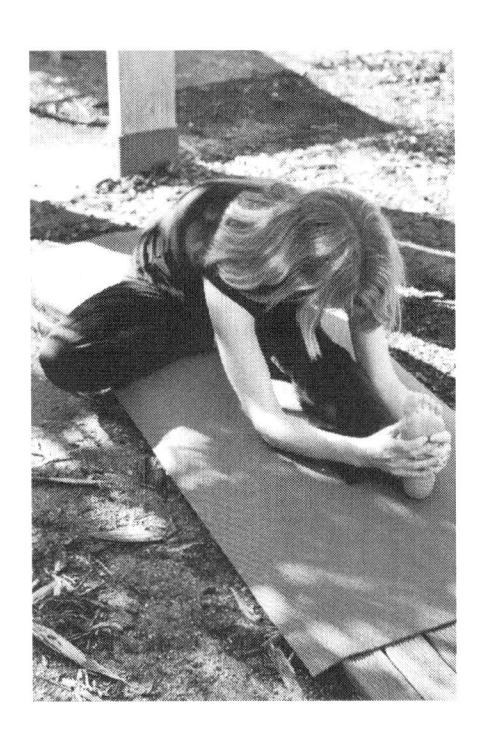

- **Upavistha Konasana (Open Angle Pose)**

    This pose has many benefits. It massages the reproductive organs, stimulates the ovaries and prostate, massages the kidneys and adrenal glands, strengthens the quadriceps while stretching the hamstrings, hips and groin, and increases circulation in the pelvic area.

    o Sitting on the ground, separate the legs into a V shape, opening only as far as is comfortable for you.
    o Flex your feet and make sure your knees are pointing straight up towards the sky.

- Press your thighs down into the ground and place your hands in front of you.
- Inhale and lift your chest, lengthening the spine, as you exhale, slowly start to walk your fingertips forward.
- Keep the spine long and move slowly with the breath, going only as far as you feel comfortable.

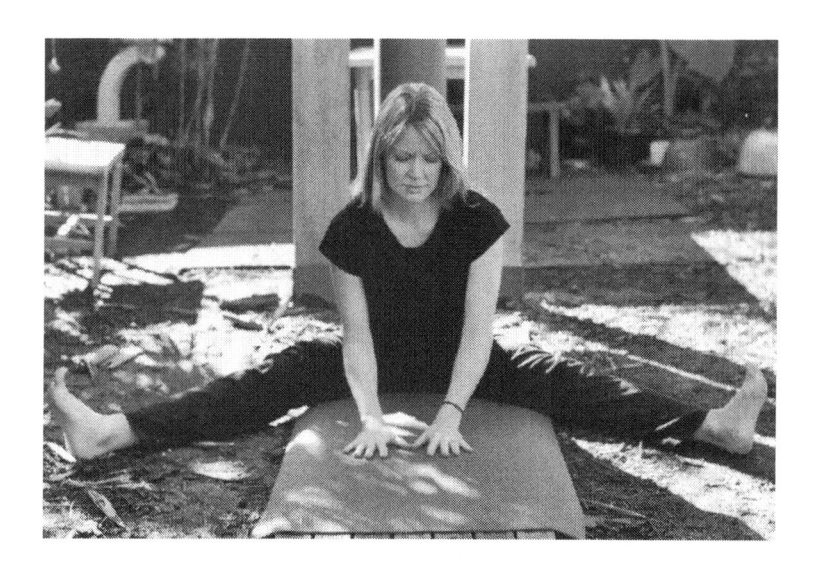

- **Parsva Upavistha Konasana (Revolved Open Angle Pose)**

    This pose is designed to improve circulation in the pelvis, to stimulate the ovaries and kidneys, and to regulate menstrual flow.

    - Sit up in Upavistha Konasana with the legs in a V shape.

- Inhale and lift the chest.
- As you exhale, turn your torso towards the right leg.
- Take another inhale, lengthening through the spine and as you exhale, release the torso over your right thigh.
- Relax the torso over the thigh and continue to breathe slowly and deeply.
- Perform the pose over your left leg as well.

Modification: If the stretch feels too intense, lay a blanket on your extended leg and rest your head and torso on the blanket.

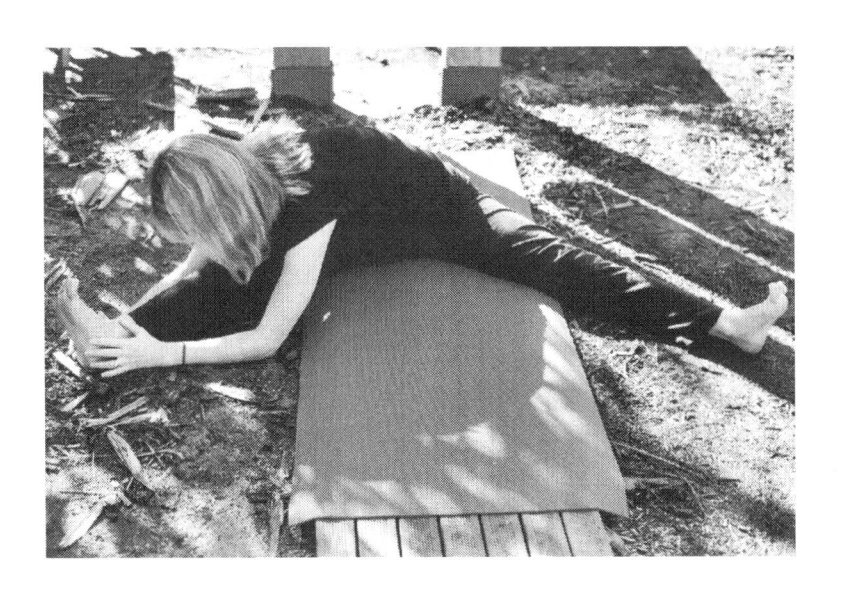

- **Setu Bandha Sarvangasana (Bridge Pose)**

This pose increases circulation in the reproductive tract and maintains and/or restores hormonal balance.

- Lie on your back with your knees bent and your feet on the floor.
- Open up your feet hip distance apart and bring them in close to your body.
- Rest your arms along your torso with the palms down.
- As you inhale, lift your hips and roll the tops of your shoulders underneath your body.
- Interlace your fingers under your lifted back and press your pinkie fingers down into the earth.
- Slightly squeeze your knees towards each other so they remain hip distance apart.
- Feel your chest opening and energy flowing through your pelvis.
- After five breaths, release your hands, come onto your toes and roll back down your spine one vertebrae at a time.
- Rest for a few breaths and then come back into the pose two more times.

Modification: If you are unable to interlace your fingers, feel free to place your hands, palms down on the ground instead. You may also rest your hips on a few stacked blankets instead of using the strength of your thighs to hold your body off of the ground.

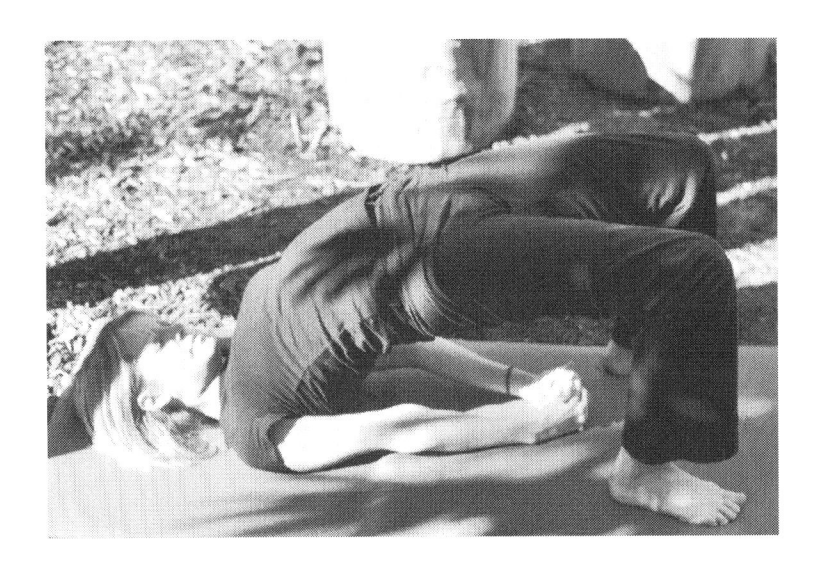

- **Supported Bridge pose**
    - o   Lie on your back with your knees bent and your feet flat on the floor.
    - o   Walk your feet as close to your buttocks as possible.
    - o   Inhale and exhale, and then slowly raise your pelvis and buttocks off the floor, while keeping your thighs and inner feet parallel.
    - o   Clasp your hands behind your back.
    - o   Hold this pose, while breathing deeply, for a minute or so.

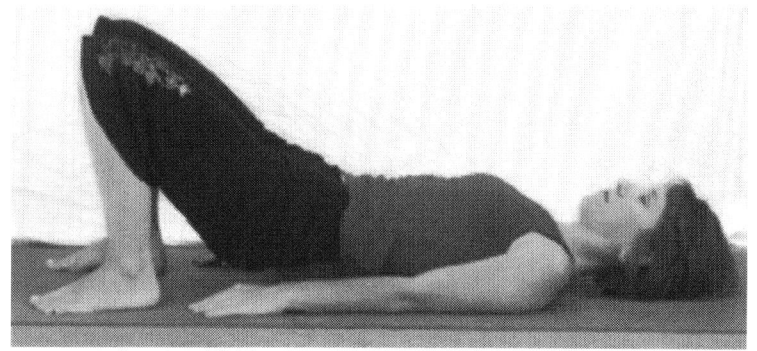

Supported Bridge   © Barry Stone

- **Yoga Nidrasana (Happy Baby Pose)**

    This pose opens the hips, massages the sexual organs, and stimulates immune function through the lymph nodes in the groin.

    - Lying on your back, place the right foot on the ground with the right knee bent.
    - Bend the left knee and take a hold of the sole of your foot with both hands.
    - Press the knee towards the ground outside of the left hip, keeping the sole of the foot pointed towards the sky with the knee bent at a 90 degree angle.
    - To deepen the stretch, straighten your right leg out on the ground.
    - On your exhale, allow any tension that is stored in pelvis and hips to melt away.
    - After a few breaths, switch sides.

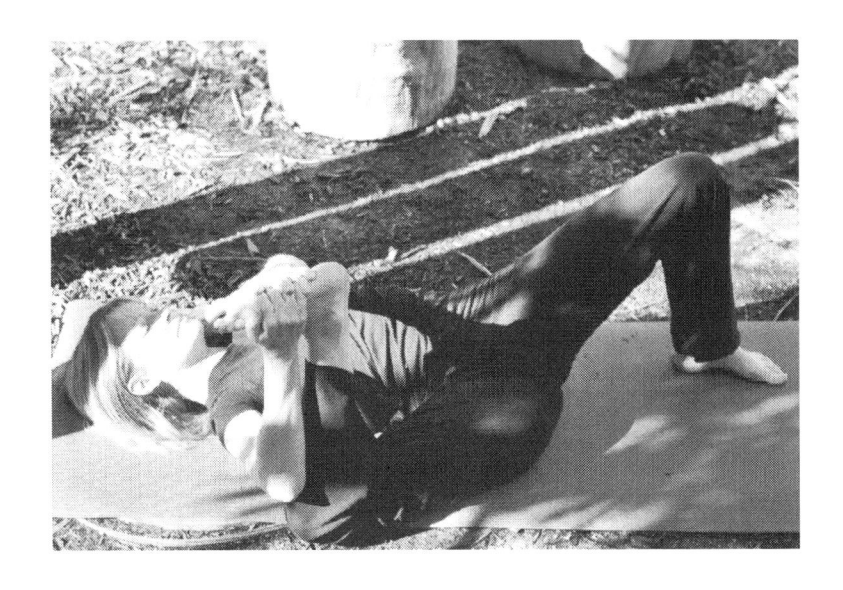

- **Supta Baddha Konasana (Reclining Bound Angle Pose)**

    This pose is designed to promote circulation in the pelvis, to open the hip joints, makes space in the pelvis and allows tension to release in the abdomen (improving digestion and elimination), to open the chest, to clear the mind, and to calm the nerves during times of stress.

    - While lying on the ground, bend your knees so the feet are on the ground close to your body.
    - Bring the feet all the way together and allow the knees to open out to the sides.
    - Tuck your pelvis so the low back is reaching towards the floor.
    - Place your arms alongside your body with the palms facing up or on your low belly.

- Elongate the back of the neck by slightly tucking the chin in towards the chest.
- Allow your body to sink into the earth, relaxing all of your muscles.
- Feel the pelvis floor and groin relaxing with every exhalation.

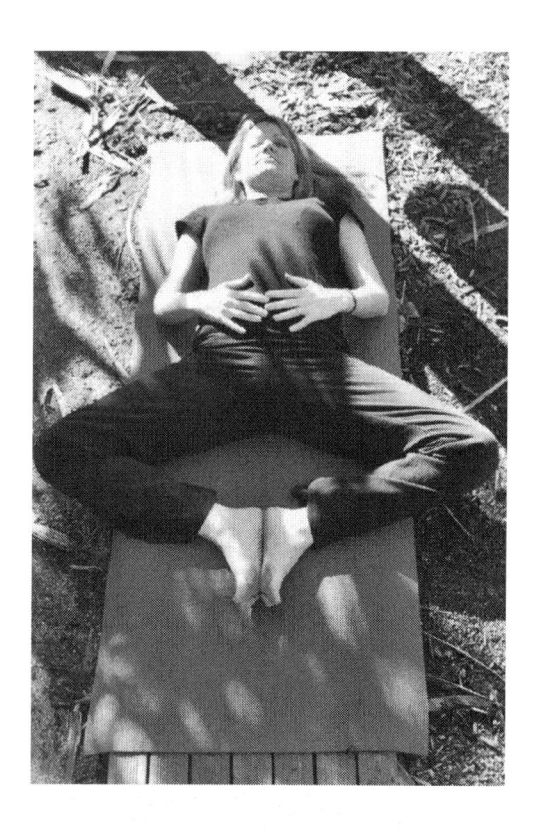

Modification: Place a blanket under each thigh for extra support if you feel any muscle tension in the legs.

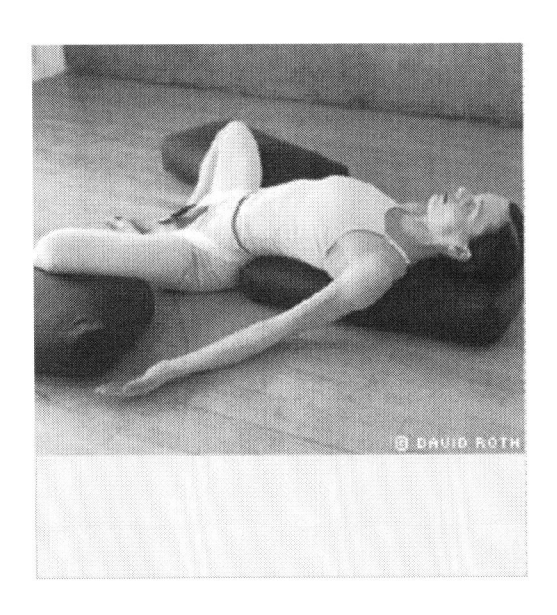

- **Viparita Karani & Variations (Legs-Up-the-Wall Pose)**

    This pose calms your nervous system, relieves fatigue, and increases blood flow to your pelvic region (do not do this pose if you are menstruating as it can interfere with your natural flow).

    o   Sit with the right side of your body next to the wall.
    o   Shift your weight onto your left hip and lower your left shoulder onto the ground so that you can bring your legs so they are resting up the wall.
    o   Scoot your rear as close to the wall as you can with the backs of your legs straight and resting against the wall.
    o   Bring your legs all the way together.

- Rest your entire torso on the ground comfortably.
- Rest your hands on your belly and bring your breath there.
- Imagine your breath bringing health and vitality to your reproductive organs.
- Close your eyes and let your body surrender into the pose.

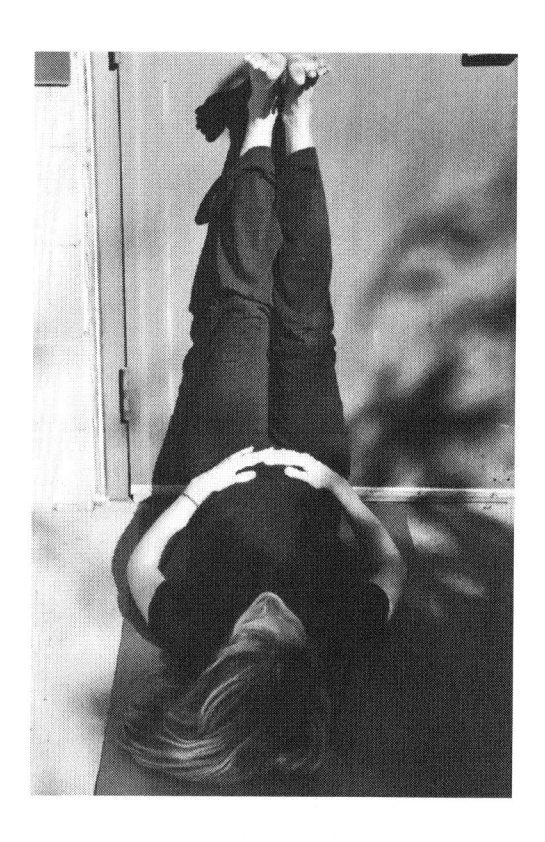

Variation: While keeping your torso the same, allow your legs to slide down the wall into a V shape.

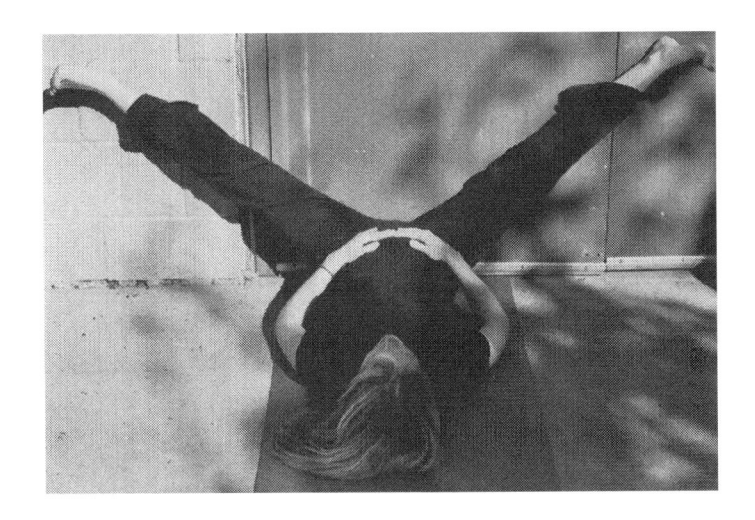

Variation: From here, bend your knees, bringing the soles of your feet together, resting your knees against the wall.

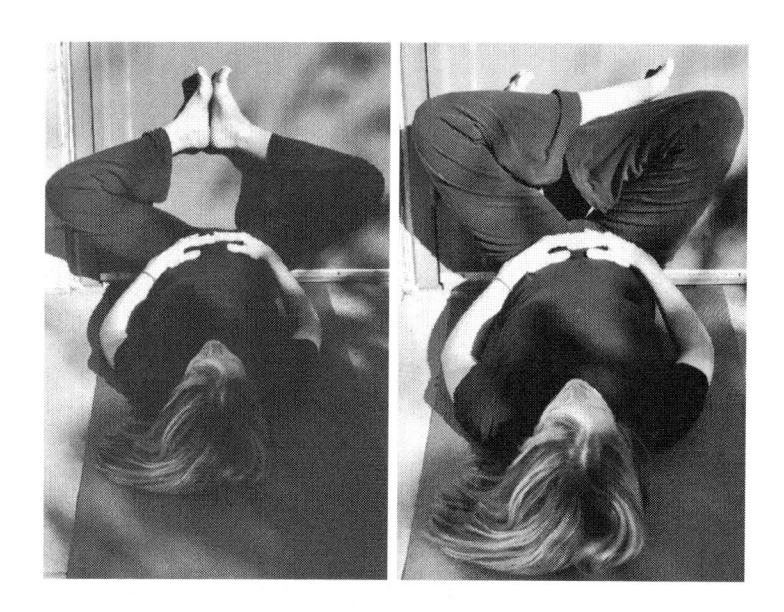

To come out of the pose, slowly slide your legs down the wall, bending your knees. Use your feet to gently push your body away from the wall.

Modification: Place a folded blanked lengthwise a couple of inches away from the wall. Rest your torso on the ground with your hips on the bolster, allowing your tailbone to dip towards the floor. If you feel discomfort in the backs of your legs, push your rear slightly away from the wall.

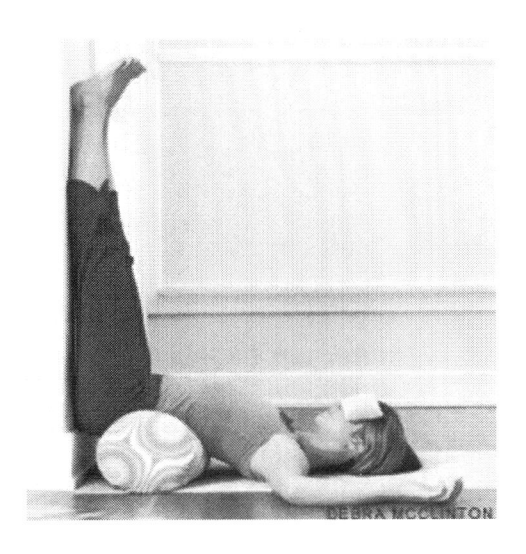

- **Savasana (Corpse Pose)**

    This pose releases and restores the entire body, quiets the mind, and relieves fatigue.

    - Lie down on the backside of you body.
    - Close your eyes and use a small towel or eye pillow to cover the eyes for deeper relaxation.
    - Separate your feet to hip distance apart and allow the toes to turn out and relax down towards the ground.
    - Bring the hands about a foot away from the body and turn your palms up, allowing your shoulders to drop towards the ground.
    - Lengthen the back of your neck on the ground so that your chin is tucked in slightly towards your chest.

- Take a moment to adjust your body so that every muscle and organ can relax as the earth easily supports every part of your body.
- Take a moment to bring some warmth to the space between your eyes.
- Allow the warmth to travel over your face and neck, spreading down into every part of your body.
- Feel as if your entire body is melting into the earth like butter, allowing all of your thoughts to dissolve.
- Stay in savasana for at least 5 minutes, but feel free to stay in the position for as long as you like.

- **When you are ready to come out of savasana**, take a few deep breaths into your belly, bringing more life and energy into your body.
- Take a moment to wiggle your fingers and toes, roll your ankles and wrists, and take any additional stretches.
- Bring your knees into your chest and roll to your side, taking a couple of breaths here.
- Use your top hand to press yourself up into a seated position and take a moment to just notice how your body and mind feels.

- o Try to maintain the sense of peace and stillness that you have created and take it with you into the rest of your day.

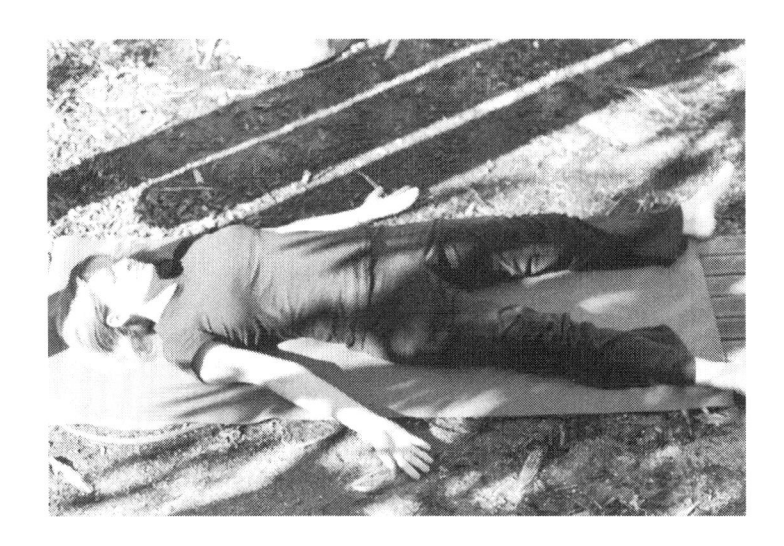

- Cobbler's Pose
    - Sit on the floor with your legs stretched out straight in front of you.
    - While inhaling, bring your feet towards your groin, and push the soles of your feet together.
    - While exhaling, slowly try to lower your knees to the ground while holding on to your toes.
    - Hold this posture, without straining your legs, for between one and five minutes.

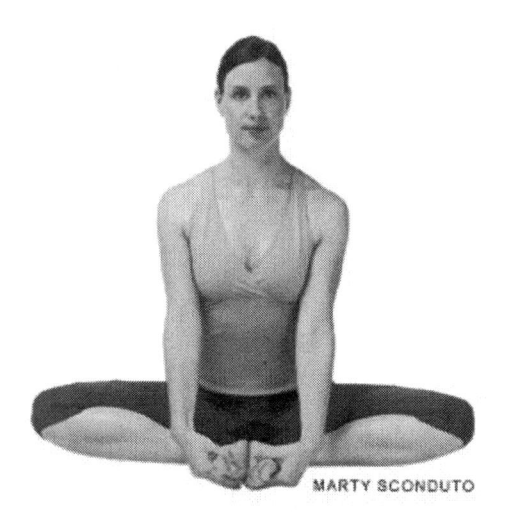

Chapter 14: Guided Imagery

Guided Imagery refers to the use of visual, kinesthetic, olfactory, taste, tactile, verbal, and auditory images in concert with relaxation techniques to promote better access to the information that our bodies store. Imagery can be used to deepen relaxation, to facilitate hypnosis, to learn more about ourselves, and to unlock *secrets* housed within the body. Sometimes the secrets are nothing more than ideas of beliefs that we have once held that maintain habits, or even, inhibit fertility.

The first exercise below provides you with an opportunity to achieve a deep relaxation and to create a space to dream and manifest. You will create a sacred space where to which you can always come, and in which you can deeply relax and honor all of your thoughts, feelings, beliefs, values and ideas.

g. Serenity Space

- Find a place to get comfortable where you can sit or lie down comfortably.
- Take a deep breath and allow your eyes to close. As they close, feel the stress and tension flowing out of your body through your arms and legs.
- As you inhale again, focus on any remaining stress or tension in your body. As you exhale, imagine yourself blowing all the stress from your body.
- Feel the tension draining from your head, through your neck and shoulders, through your back and torso, through your pelvis, legs, and arms and out your fingers and toes.
- As you relax, breathe comfortably, in and out, allowing your attention to remain on your breath. The more comfortable you become, the more relaxed you are.
- As you relax, allow yourself to feel the weightlessness that you can sometimes feel before drifting off to sleep.
- Imagine that a wonderful, warm fog begins to envelope you. The fog is warm, but not hot, and cool, but not cold. It is perfectly safe, secure and comforting in this fog.
- Feel yourself gently propelled forward through the fog into a clearing.
- As you come into the clearing, see before you the most beautiful place you have ever seen, whether real or imagined.

- Take in all the sights, sounds, and smells in this place. Allow all of your senses to experience the beauty and comfort of this place.
- Walk freely and comfortably until you find a perfect spot to relax and restore yourself.

h. Inner Advisor

When you are ready to proceed, you are encouraged to become acquainted with the wisest, most compassionate, part of yourself. We refer to this part of you as your *Inner Advisor*.

- Walk comfortably here until you find a place to relax- whether seated or reclining.
- When you are able to sit or lie down, take a deep breath and imagine what it would be like if you could know how to improve your life and your relationship. Imagine if you could know yourself well enough to remove any obstacles to beginning your family.
- When you are ready, you can ask your Inner Advisor to join you in this beautiful place. The Inner Advisor is the wisest, most competent and nurturant part of you. It may take any form it chooses- it may be a person, animal, shape, sound, or even a feeling. The Inner Advisor will come to you as soon as you invite it to do so.
- When your Advisor appears, thank your Advisor for coming to you. Invite your

Advisor to communicate with you in a way that will be easy for you to understand.

➢ This is an opportunity for you to ask questions that have not been answered yet. This is also an opportunity for your advisor to give you messages and instructions about you might improve your life.

➢ Consider what questions you might like to ask.

➢ Some common questions include:

- o "What do I need to do differently to improve my stress level?"
- o "What have I not heard that I need to hear?"
- o "What messages am I not attending to?"
- o "How can I be more welcoming to my family and any souls that may want to join us?"
- o "What skills do I need to learn?"

➢ As you feel able, pose these questions to your Advisor.

➢ Listen with your ears, eyes, mind, and spirit. Advisors do not always communicate verbally, but everyone has the ability to experience the answers provided by their Advisor.

➢ When you feel satisfied with this first exchange with your Advisor, thank your Advisor for coming. Ask your Advisor how you will be able to make contact again, and if there is "homework" that you need to do before your next exchange.

- When your Advisor is ready, s/he will exit.
- Take a deep breath and walk towards the fog at the edge of the clearing. As you enter the fog, feel again the comfort and security there. Allow yourself to be enveloped, feeling the relaxation blanket you.
- As we count back from 5 to 1, you will feel refreshed, and clear about what you have learned.
- At 5 you will begin to feel the chair or ground beneath you. At 4 you will become more aware of those around you.
- At 3 you will begin to hear the sounds of the room. At 2 you will take a deep breath and prepare to be back in the room. And, at 1, you will allow your eyes to flicker open.

How was the experience for you?

_____

_____

_____

_____

_____

_____

_____

_____

_____

_____

What form did your Inner Advisor take?

_____

_____

_____

_____

_____

How did your Advisor communicate with you?

_____

_____

_____

_____

What did you learn?

What messages did you receive?

_____

_____

_____

_____

_____

_____

_____

What skills do you need to acquire?

_____

_____

_____

_____

_____

How will you connect with your Advisor again?

_____

_____

_____

_____

_____

_____

_____

How did this experience compare to the other exercises?

_____

_____

_____

_____

_____

_____

_____

_____

Once you have learned how to deepen the relationship with yourself, there is no limit to what you can learn. The Inner Advisor relaxation exercise allows you to connect to the wisest part of yourself, but may not answer specific questions about your body and its function.

i. Healing from Within

Often, couples that desire to improve chances for pregnancy want to know if there are problems with their bodies and organs that are as yet unknown. Sometimes, women feel as if something is getting in the way of conception, even though the OB says that no physical problems exist.

These messages are best gleaned from interacting directly with the part of the body that may be experiencing difficulties. While it may be an unusual practice for you, learning to speak and *listen to* specific parts of your body can be enlightening and life-changing!

➢ Find yourself a comfortable place.

➢ Breathe deeply and allow your eyes to close.

➢ As you inhale, focus on any tension you may have. As you exhale, allow all the stress to exit your body, leaving you feeling completely relaxed.

➢ With your next deep breath, imagine that you are going to enter your body, flashlight in hand from the crown at the top of your head.

➢ Travel down through your interior until you reach a place where you can rest for a moment.

➢ Ask your body which part would like to communicate with you.

➢ Travel to that part of the body. When you have reached this area, shine your light around. Examine this area. Is it filled with light or is it dark? Is it pleasant, or has it been neglected or abused? How does it seem?

➢ Give this area or organ a voice and allow it to communicate directly with you.

➢ What questions would you ask of this part?

➢ What would you like to learn from this part?

➢ As we count back from 5 to 1, you will feel refreshed, and clear about what you have learned.

➢ At 5 you will begin to feel the chair or ground beneath you. At 4 you will become more aware of those around you.

➢ At 3 you will begin to hear the sounds of the room. At 2 you will take a deep breath and prepare to be back in the room. And, at 1, you will allow your eyes to flicker open.

How was the experience for you?

_____

_____

_____

_____

_____

What body parts made themselves known?

_____

_____

_____

_____

_____

What did these parts have to say?

What did you learn?

How can you apply what you experienced so that your body feels more respected, can function more optimally, and can conceive and maintain a pregnancy?

Chapter 15: Cognitive Concepts for Conception

Right from the very beginning of this process, you came to recognize that your fertility hinges on how and what you think and believe. You considered the impacts of your beliefs on your fertility, but perhaps we need to take it a step further. It may be necessary to not only consider what you think, but also *why* you think things happen. This is referred to as your *locus of control*.

j. Locus of Control

People either see themselves as in control of what happens to them (and also in control of the solutions they create), or as victims of external elements around them.

In addition, people are either optimistic within that locus of control (they believe that things will be manageable and have a positive end) or they are pessimistic or negativistic in their locus of control (they believe that things are more likely to result in consequences that do not favor them).

On following scale below, where do you fall in terms of your locus of control?

0_____100

External locus   *Internal locus*

"Things happen to me"   *"I make things happen"*

And how do you perceive yourself on the continuum between optimism and pessimism?

0_____100

Pessimism

Optimism

"Things won't work out"   "Things will work out for the best"

k. **Beliefs about Conception, Pregnancy & Family**

Take some time to make note below of specific positive or negative beliefs that you have about conception, pregnancy, and family.

Beliefs about Conception:

_____

_____

_____

_____

_____

_____

_____

_____

Beliefs about Pregnancy:

_____

_____

_____

_____

_____

_____

_____

Beliefs about Family:

_____

_____

_____

_____

_____

_____

_____

1. Cognitive Distortions: Sabotaging Self-talk

Cognitive distortions refer to the way we twist our thinking to create perception or interpretation of what has actually been said to us. The end result is typically negative, leading us to be victims of our own misguided thought processes.

By becoming more aware of the way we distort our thoughts, we can *unlearn* this bad habit and shift to healthier ways of thinking.

Which of these common cognitive distortions do you regularly use?

- ☐ Filtering
- ☐ All or nothing thinking
- ☐ Overgeneralization
- ☐ Mindreading
- ☐ Catastrophizing
- ☐ Personalization
- ☐ Control Fallacies
- ☐ Fallacy of Fairness
- ☐ Blaming
- ☐ Shoulds
- ☐ Emotional Reasoning
- ☐ Fallacy of Change

- ☐ Global labeling
- ☐ Being right
- ☐ Heaven's Reward Fallacy

What are some of the distortions that you believe your partner uses?

_____

_____

_____

_____

_____

_____

How do these distortions get in the way in the relationship?

_____

_____

_____

_____

How could these distortions inhibit conception and healthy pregnancy?

m. Altering Self-Talk: Using The Thought Log

Self-talk can be described as the voice or voices in our head, our "old tapes" or internal narrative. Self-talk is the way that we talk to ourselves about the choices we are making and their impact on our lives. Self-talk can be positive or negative, depending on how we feel about things.

Is there negative self-talk that fills your head?

___

___

___

___

___

___

Where did it come from?

___

___

___

___

If you peel back the layers of time, whose voice fills your head? (We have discovered that while the voices sound like our own from first glance, if we track them back in time, they are often the negative or critical voices of our parents, coaches, or teachers).

Using the chart below, describe a situation that didn't go so well. After you've written a description, identify all of the feelings you had in response to the situation.

Altering Self-talk

Situation	Feelings	Rate the feelings	Thoughts	Healthier thoughts	Feelings	Re-Rate the feelings

Rate the feelings on a scale from 0-100, with 100 representing the most intense feeling you could have.

Identify the self-talk or thoughts that ran through your head during the situation. If you can, identify the thoughts that ran beneath those thoughts.

What are the negative, core or "hot" thoughts that may have driven your negative behavioral response?

_____

_____

_____

_____

_____

_____

_____

_____

After identifying your unreasonable thoughts, generate healthier, or more reasonable thoughts to replace the negative or unreasonable thoughts. This new self-talk is based on resolving the cognitive distortions. For instance, a statement such as "Everyone will know that I'm not a good mother" might be altered to "There is no evidence that I'm a bad mother."

After all of the unhealthy thoughts have been addressed, identify all of your feelings about the situation now. After you've listed the feelings, re-rate the feelings, using a range from 0-100, with 100 being the most intense experience of the feeling.

Most of us discover that by changing our thoughts from negative to positive, or from unhealthy to healthy, our feelings also change. Many people report significant decreases in negative or uncomfortable feelings and increases in positive feelings (such as empowered, confident, and strong).

By using these techniques to identify thoughts, beliefs, and negative self-talk about conception, pregnancy, and family, you increase your chances for healthy conception and pregnancy.

Experience the power of positive thinking!

Chapter 16: Fertility & Feelings

n. Listening In – Getting Tuned in and Turned on!

The most important part of listening to your partner, is learning first, to listen to yourself. "Listening in" is simply a tool to help you get "into it" or I-N-T-U-I-T.

Intuition is nothing more than listening at a greater intensity than you might normally use.

Often, mothers believe that they "maternal instinct"- or a basic knowingness about what their children want or need. Others may refer to have a "gut feeling" about things. Reporters and brokers often work on the basis of "hunches". All of those terms describe *ways in which we get i-n-t-u-i-t*.

When we get "into" our bodies and our spirits, we arm ourselves with a world of information that we may otherwise dismiss or ignore. When it comes to feelings, the best way to ensure that your feelings don't negatively impact your body, is to really *know* what those feelings are.

When you are experiencing emotion, what does it feel like?

___

___

___

___

___

___

When I am happy, I feel this way in my body:

___

___

___

___

___

___

When I am angry, I feel this way in my body:

_____

_____

_____

_____

_____

_____

_____

_____

0. Clearing the Decks

    In order to clearly identify and understand our feelings and those of our partners and friends, it is important that we have an awareness about our emotional comfort level. Often, when we are disturbed by an emotion, we will avoid or suppress it. Emotions can be pushed below the surface where they can begin to damage us, *and we might not even know it!*

    How does this work for you?

☐ I tune out to some of my feelings
☐ I tune in to my feelings

If you tune out, what feelings have been gnawing away at you beneath the surface?

☐ angry
☐ anxious
☐ apologetic
☐ apprehensive
☐ ashamed
☐ awkward
☐ bitter
☐ brave
☐ confused
☐ contemptuous
☐ defeated
☐ depressed
☐ deprived
☐ desperate
☐ devastated
☐ disappointed
☐ discouraged
☐ disgusted
☐ distrustful
☐ embarrassed
☐ envious
☐ excited
☐ excluded
☐ fearful
☐ foolish
☐ frustrated

- ☐ fulfilled
- ☐ furious
- ☐ grateful
- ☐ guilty
- ☐ happy
- ☐ helpless
- ☐ helpless
- ☐ hopeless
- ☐ horrified
- ☐ hostile
- ☐ humiliated
- ☐ hurt
- ☐ ignored
- ☐ impatient
- ☐ inadequate
- ☐ incompetent
- ☐ inferior
- ☐ inhibited
- ☐ inhibited
- ☐ insecure
- ☐ irritated
- ☐ isolated
- ☐ jealous
- ☐ joyful
- ☐ left out
- ☐ lonely
- ☐ loveable
- ☐ miserable
- ☐ out-of-control
- ☐ outraged
- ☐ overwhelmed
- ☐ panicky
- ☐ pressured

- ☐ proud
- ☐ provoked
- ☐ rejected
- ☐ relaxed
- ☐ relieved
- ☐ remorseful
- ☐ resentful
- ☐ sad
- ☐ secure
- ☐ self-conscious
- ☐ shy
- ☐ sorry
- ☐ stubborn
- ☐ stuck
- ☐ stupid
- ☐ threatened
- ☐ touchy
- ☐ trapped
- ☐ troubled
- ☐ unappreciated
- ☐ unattractive
- ☐ uncertain
- ☐ uncomfortable
- ☐ understood
- ☐ uneasy
- ☐ untrustworthy
- ☐ unworthy
- ☐ uptight
- ☐ used
- ☐ useless
- ☐ victimized
- ☐ vulnerable
- ☐ vulnerable

☐ worried

p. Feelings associated with Conception & Pregnancy

Knowing that feelings can be associated with any and all parts of our lives, are there any feelings about conception, pregnancy or parenthood that are too difficult to manage in your waking day? If so, what happens to those feelings?

Feelings that I may have about conception and pregnancy, but may not spend time reviewing or processing include:

_____

_____

_____

_____

_____

_____

_____

_____

It is possible to know oneself well enough to have clear and conscious awareness of those feelings which prove to be obstacles to our fertility. However, sometimes those feelings reside outside of our awareness and need to be invited into our consciousness. The following is an exercise that can help you gain clarity about the feelings you may have that could inhibit conception and pregnancy.

- Find a comfortable spot that will facilitate your relaxation.
- Breathe deeply a few times so that you can let your eyes close, and your mind turn inwards.
- Breathe deeply so that oxygen floods all of your muscles and brings deep relaxation and comfort to your entire body.
- Breathe deeply again and imagine washing away everything that belongs to everyone else, whether that is work, worry, or wishes.
- Now, bring your focus to your desire to start new life. Imagine what life would be like if you were able to create and conceive.
- What feeling courses through your body? Likely, there are many feelings! What are they?
- Bring your awareness to all of the feelings that you are experiencing- are these familiar? Are they comfortable? Are they

satisfying? What do these feelings tell you? What messages come from these feelings?

➤ If your Inner Advisor were to speak with you about these feelings, what would the Advisor say?

➤ When you have a sense of these feelings, allow yourself to breathe deeply and let go of the intensity of these feelings. Experience the feelings as if they were muted- you can still feel them, but they are quieter and less intrusive now.

➤ With the next deep breath, become aware of your surroundings, and allow your eyes to flutter open.

What did you find?

_____

_____

_____

_____

_____

_____

_____

_____

_____

What feelings might inhibit new life?

What feelings support you on your journey?

q. It Takes Two to Tango – Getting Tuned into your Partner

Whether or not you inhibit or tune out emotion, the ability to conceive actually takes two- meaning that stagnant emotion, FOR EITHER OF YOU, can inhibit this process. That means that you and your partner must be responsible enough to both experience and EXPRESS your emotions.

The following exercise can help you get a better sense of your partner's feelings.

- In order to get INTUIT, breathe deeply and wash your own story away.
- Then imagine breathing in your partner and their story.
- Allow yourself to sample any feelings that come in as you breathe.
- As soon as you experience the feeling, let it go- much like reading a piece of someone's mail, then handing it back to them.
- Breathe deeply again, and imagine pulling away from your partner, back into your own space.

What was your experience like?

What were the feelings that you experienced with your partner?

Were there any stories there? What were they?

How did you feel about what you found?

Chapter 17: Listening to your Lover

1. Receiving Messages: What do you *really* hear?

    The following is a questionnaire that may help you to evaluate your listening skills. Try to be as honest as you can, then review the results and determine how this may impact communications with your partner, friends, family, and fertility team.

Receiving Messages

Reprinted with permission from Lussier, R. N. (1990). *Human Relations in Organization: A Skill-building Approach.* Columbus, OH: Irwin Professional Publishing (McGraw-Hill).

When asked, "are you a good listener?" most people say yes. In reality, 75 percent of what people hear they hear imprecisely and 75 percent of what they hear accurately they forget within three weeks. [43] In other words, most people are poor listeners.

Select the response that best describes the frequency of your actual behavior. Place the letters A, U, F, O or S on the line before each of the 15 statements.

Almost always   Usually   Frequently   Occasionally   Seldom

    A   U   F   O
    S

1. ____ I like to listen to people talk. I encourage them to talk by showing interest, by smiling and nodding, etc.

2. ____ I pay closer attention to speakers who are more interesting or similar to me.

3. ____ I evaluate the speaker's words and nonverbal communication ability as they talk.

4. ____ I avoid distractions; if it's noisy, I suggest moving to a quiet spot, etc.

5. ____ When people interrupt me to talk, I put what I was doing out of sight and mind and give them my complete attention.

6. ____ When people are talking I allow them time to finish. I do not interrupt, anticipate what they are going to say, or jump to conclusions.

7. ____ I tune people out who do not agree with my views.

8. ____ While the other person is talking or the professor is lecturing, my mind wanders to personal topics.

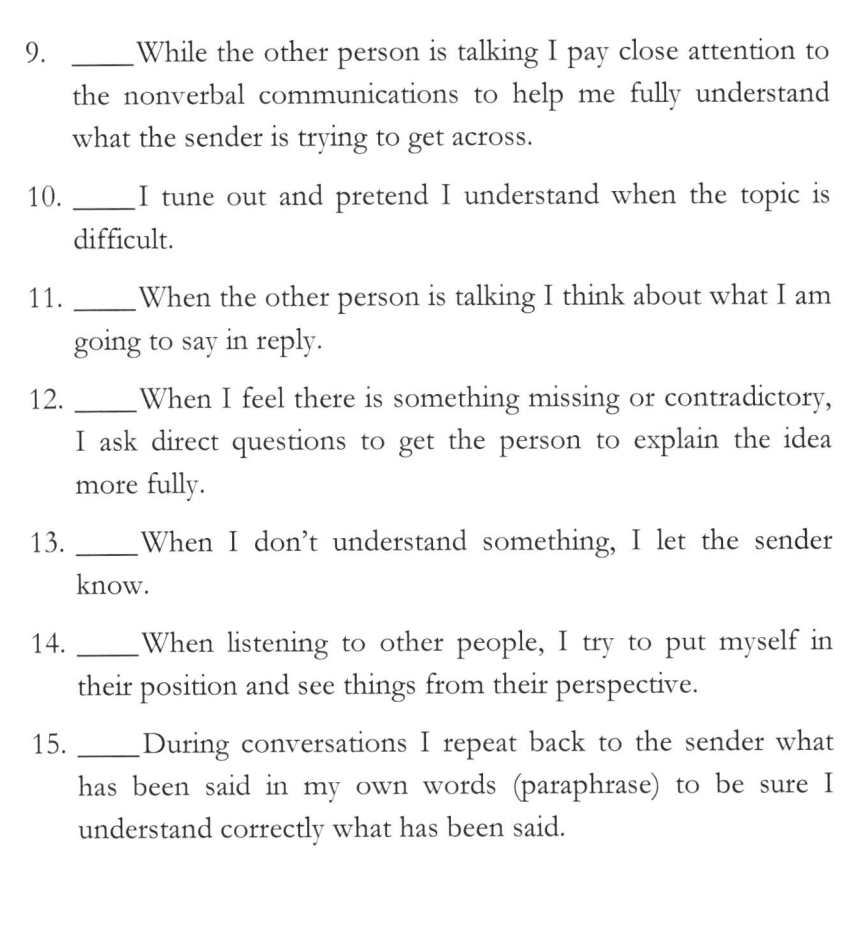

9. ____While the other person is talking I pay close attention to the nonverbal communications to help me fully understand what the sender is trying to get across.

10. ____I tune out and pretend I understand when the topic is difficult.

11. ____When the other person is talking I think about what I am going to say in reply.

12. ____When I feel there is something missing or contradictory, I ask direct questions to get the person to explain the idea more fully.

13. ____When I don't understand something, I let the sender know.

14. ____When listening to other people, I try to put myself in their position and see things from their perspective.

15. ____During conversations I repeat back to the sender what has been said in my own words (paraphrase) to be sure I understand correctly what has been said.

If you were to have people to whom you talk regularly answer these questions about you, would they have the same responses that you selected? Have friends fill out the questions for you and compare answers.

To determine your score, give yourself 5 points for each A, 4 for each U, 3 for each F, 2 for each O, and 1 for each S for statements 1, 4, 5, 6, 9, 12, 13, 14, and 15. Place the numbers on the line to your response letter. For items 2, 3, 7, 8, 10, and 11 the score reverses: 5 points for each S, 4 for each O, 3 for each F, 2 for each U and 1 for each A.

Place these score numbers on the lines next to the response letters.

Now add your total number of points. Your score should be between 15 and 75.

Place your score here and on the continuum below. _____

Poor listener   15_ _ _ 25 _ _ _ 35 _ _ _ 45 _ _ _ 55 _ _ _ 65 _ _ _ 75 Good listener

Generally, the higher your score, the better your listening skills.

s. Sensory Modalities: How do you hear?

Sensory modalities are the ways in which we hear and communicate with others. Modalities include:

1. Verbal
2. Visual
3. Auditory
4. Olfactory
5. Taste
6. Kinesthetics

Which do you use primarily? Secondarily?

Are there those that you don't use well?

Which does your partner use?

Are their times that you or your partner use one modality more than another?

_____

_____

_____

_____

Do you ever feel as if you're speaking two different languages? If so, this may be a sign that you are experiencing a sensory mismatch.

What would it take for you to learn your partner's language? What would it require for your partner to learn to communicate in your sensory modality?

_____

_____

_____

_____

_____

_____

_____

_____

t. Effective Listening

Once we have a grasp of *how* we listen, we must learn to apply effective listening skills. For optimal results when listening, it is important to follow a few guidelines:

1. Use good basic listening habits:

    ➤ *How well do you pay attention?*

    _____

    _____

    _____

    _____

    _____

    _____

    _____

➢ *Do you listen to the whole message?*

_____

_____

_____

_____

_____

➢ *Are you able to hear the message before evaluating or judging it?*

_____

_____

_____

_____

➢ *Do you paraphrase what you've heard for verification of the message?*

_____

_____

_____
_____
_____

2. Avoid bad listening habits

   > *Are you guilty of using "selective attention"?*

   _____
   _____
   _____
   _____
   _____

   > *Do you sometimes find yourself "pseudolistening"?*

   _____
   _____
   _____

➢ *Do you ever listen without hearing?*

➢ *Do you interrupt?*

➢ *Do you ever disclose too much too soon?*

3. Define the issue

   ➢ *Can you identify why the issue is being addressed now?*

   ➢ *Has this issue been addressed before?*

➤ *If so, was the issue resolved before? If so, how was it resolved?*

4. Use passive listening skills at first:

➤ *Are you willing to let your partner do the talking*

➢ *Can you attend to how your partner is communicating in addition to what is being said?*

___

➢ *Can you keep your opinions to yourself for now?*

___

➢ *Are you able to empathize with your partner?*

_____

_____

_____

5. Use active listening skills after the issue has been reviewed

   > *Were you able to paraphrase? Clarify? Personalize?*

_____

_____

_____

_____

u. Assertive Communication: Speaking to be heard

Assertive communication is a direct and honest expression of your desires which is considerate of both your own needs and desires and those of your partner's.

When you communicate, are you open, honest, and direct?

Are you respectful or both yourself and others?

Do you feel overwhelming anxiety or guilt?

There are many styles of communicating, including passive, aggressive, passive-aggressive, and assertive. Which style best describes how you communicate?

_____

_____

_____

_____

What impact does this have on how you and your partner communicate?

_____

_____

_____

_____

_____

_____

_____

How does this impact the communication you have with your fertility team?

_____

_____

_____

_____

_____

_____

_____

_____

v. Rights I Have

It is important that we all recognize the rights that we have. Unfortunately, we do not always experience our lives, or communicate as if we have these rights. Identify which of these rights you perceive, and with whom.

Rights I Have

On a scale of 1 to 5, rate each right as it applies to your relationship with self, partner, fertility team, and others

1	2	3	4	5
Never		*Occasionally*		*Always*

Right	with Self	with Partner	with Team	with Others
1. I have the right to change my mind.				
2. I have the right to say "no!"				
3. I have the right to ask for favors.				
4. I have the right to ask for emotional support.				
5. I have the right to spend time doing what I want to do.				
6. I have the right to disagree with others.				
7. I have the right to be treated with respect.				
8. I have the right to make my own decisions.				
9. I have the right to reject others' advice or suggestions.				
10. I have the right to say "yes!" to things I want to do.				
11. I have the right to take a vacation or day off.				
12. I have the right to put my needs and wants ahead of those of others.				
13. I have the right to express my feelings.				

14. I have the right to compliment myself.
15. I have the right to accept or reject others' criticisms of me.
16. I have the right to accept others' compliments of me.
17. I have the right to be close to others.
18. I have the right to be physically and emotionally healthy.
19. I have the right to be sexually fulfilled.
20. I have the right to desire great things.

In examining your responses, what did you learn about yourself?

_____

_____

_____

_____

_____

Are there rights which you do not maintain, that negatively impact your relationships?

_____

_____

_____

_____

_____

i. The Assertive Communication Template

Speaking assertively is not always easy for some of us, especially in highly conflicted situations. Use the template below to practice developing assertive statements!

➢ Describe

  o When you…

  _____
  _____
  _____
  _____
  _____

➢ Express

  o I feel…

  _____
  _____
  _____
  _____

- Specify
  - I want… would like… would appreciate…

  _____
  _____
  _____
  _____
  _____
  _____
  _____
  _____

- Consequences
  - If you do… (state the reward)

  _____
  _____
  _____
  _____
  _____
  _____
  _____
  _____
  _____

➢ If you don't (state the action you will carry out)

_____
_____
_____
_____
_____
_____
_____
_____
_____
_____
_____

Chapter 18: Old Baggage I Carry

In order to best avoid carrying old baggage into new relationships, it is important to manage the challenges as they present. Or, alternatively, if you've found yourself burdened by overfull emotional suitcases, attend to the issues as soon as you become aware of them!

Some of the challenges that life may present include the following circumstances:

- [ ] Parental divorce
- [ ] Loss of a parent or grandparent
- [ ] Geographic moves
- [ ] Loss or absence of friendships
- [ ] Emotional or psychological abuse
- [ ] Verbal abuse
- [ ] Physical abuse

- [ ] Sexual abuse or trauma
- [ ] Accidents
- [ ] Being a victim of crime
- [ ] Loss of relationship
- [ ] Divorce
- [ ] Custody disputes
- [ ] Birth or death of a child
- [ ] Infertility
- [ ] Financial distress
- [ ] Legal problems
- [ ] Incarceration
- [ ] Chronic or terminal illness
- [ ] Surgical alterations or reconstruction
- [ ] Loss of job or career change

What, if any, are challenges that you have experienced?

Check all that apply to you, in the present or the past.

Have you allowed yourself time to experience, express, and find closure with these issues?

_____

_____

Do you carry any of these issues around as baggage?

If you do, what's in the baggage?

For the baggage that you carry, what do you need to do in order to put it down and move forward with your new reality?

_____
_____
_____
_____
_____
_____
_____
_____
_____
_____
_____
_____

Chapter 19: Commitment to Love: Agreement for the NOW, as well as for the Future

Find a quiet place in which you are safe to think about your relationship.

Which of the following relationship components are already present in your relationship?

- ☐ Individuality
- ☐ Acceptance (of self and others)
- ☐ Honesty
- ☐ Respect
- ☐ Consideration
- ☐ Communication & Understanding
- ☐ Trust
- ☐ Vulnerability

☐ Mutual Sexual Interaction
☐ Empathy
☐ Compassion
☐ Congruence

Which are missing?

_____
_____
_____
_____
_____
_____
_____

Have any of them been particularly difficult for you to achieve?

_____
_____
_____

Identify the components that you would like to work on with your partner.

As you come to closure with this workbook, and with this journey, recommitment to your relationship can be a wonderful way to mark this passage. Try writing your own recommitment ceremony, or consider the ceremony below as a way to open this next chapter of your life:

Love is the eternal and divine force of life; the mirror in which we mortal humans may see the infinite expressions of God. Love is the power that allows us to face fear, challenges and uncertainty with courage and faith. We call upon Love to bless this gathering, and to shine in our hearts as we affirm our love for one another.

We come together not to mark the start of a relationship, but to recognize, as a community of love, a bond that already exists. This marriage is one expression of the many varieties of love.

We live in a world of joy and fear. We search for meaning and strength in seeming disorder. We discover the truest guideline to our quest when we realize Love in all its magnitudes.

In recommitment, we perform an act of faith. This faith can grow and mature and endure, but only if we both determine to make it so. A lasting and growing love is never guaranteed by any ceremony.

If we claim the foundation of our union to be the love we have for one another, not just at this moment, but for all the days ahead, then we can cherish the hopes and dreams that bring us here today.

We resolve that our love will never be blotted out by the commonplace, shaken by fears, nor obscured by the ordinary in life.

Let us remember that giving of ourselves in love can be difficult.

We must learn to give of love without total submission of ourselves, and yet without condition.

Therefore, in our giving, may we give our joy, our sadness, our interest, our understanding, our knowledge and all expressions that make up life. But in this giving, we will remember to preserve our identities, our integrity, and our individualities.

This is the challenge of love within marriage.

To one another, you may desire to say:

I commit my life to our partnership in marriage. I promise to comfort you. I promise to encourage you in all ways of life. I promise to express my thoughts and feelings to you. I promise to listen to you in times of joy and in times of sorrow.

I love you, and you are my closest friend. Will you let me share my life and all that I am with you?

Chapter 20: Resources for Family Alternatives

a) Surrogacy

   1. Why are you considering surrogacy?

   _____

   _____

   _____

   _____

   _____

   _____

   _____

   _____

2. Are you considering using a:

    a. gestational surrogate? _____

    b. traditional surrogate? _____

3. Is your partner committed to this plan?

_____

_____

4. Who is the driver of the surrogacy plan?
   - ☐ Me (definitely)
   - ☐ Me (a little bit more than my spouse)
   - ☐ My spouse/partner (definitely)
   - ☐ My spouse/partner (a little bit more)
   - ☐ Both want to adopt about the same

5. Will this driver/driven dynamic cause conflict in your relationship?

_____

_____

_____

_____

_____

_____

_____

_____

_____

6. What are the issues?

_____

_____

_____

_____

_____

_____

_____

_____

b) Adoption

In order to determine if adoption is right for you, spend some time considering the following questions. When you've explored the questions and generated answers, ask your partner to do the same. When you have both completed the process, share your answers with one another.

1. Why do you want to adopt?

_____

_____

_____

_____

_____

_____

_____

2. On a scale of 1 to 10, with 10 being the highest, how badly do you want to adopt?

_____

3. Who is the driver of wanting this adoption? Will this cause conflict?
    - o   Me (definitely)
    - o   Me (a little bit more than my spouse)
    - o   My spouse/partner (definitely)
    - o   My spouse/partner (a little bit more)
    - o   Both want to adopt about the same

4. Will this driver/driven dynamic cause conflict in your relationship?

5. What age child would you prefer to adopt? (Underline the preferred age, and circle all ages you would be willing to consider.)

- o Newborn (under six months)
- o Infant (newborn to 2)
- o Preschooler (3 to 5)
- o Primary school (6 to 10)
- o Middle school (11 to 14)
- o High school (15 to 18)

6. How firm are you on the age selected above?

_____

_____

_____

_____

_____

_____

7. Which of the following disabilities would you be willing to consider in an adoptive child? (Select all that you would consider)

- ☐ Drug exposed (occasional)
- ☐ Deafness
- ☐ Mild or medically correctable condition
- ☐ No drugs or alcohol considered
- ☐ Non-correctable (cerebral palsy, retardation etc.)
- ☐ Alcohol exposed (occasional)
- ☐ Alcohol exposed (frequent)
- ☐ Smoking exposed
- ☐ Emotional/mental disorders in family
- ☐ Emotional/mental disorders in child
- ☐ Premature birth
- ☐ Multiple birth
- ☐ Club foot

- ☐ Cleft pallet or lip
- ☐ Downs Syndrome
- ☐ Epilepsy in child
- ☐ Epilepsy in family
- ☐ Blindness
- ☐ Diabetes in child
- ☐ Diabetes in family
- ☐ Conceived through rape
- ☐ Conceived through incest
- ☐ Nothing known about father
- ☐ Nothing known about mother
- ☐ Sibling group

8. Which of the following racial heritages would you be willing to consider in an adoptive child? (Select all that apply)

- ☐ Any Child
- ☐ Arab/Middle Eastern
- ☐ Asian
- ☐ African American
- ☐ Caucasian
- ☐ Caucasian/Asian
- ☐ Caucasian/African American
- ☐ European
- ☐ Caucasian/Hispanic
- ☐ Caucasian/Native American

- ☐ Eastern European/Slavic/Russian
- ☐ Hispanic or South/Central American
- ☐ Mediterranean
- ☐ Middle Eastern
- ☐ Multi-Racial
- ☐ Native American (American Indian)
- ☐ Pacific Islander

9. Which gender would you prefer in your child?
    - ☐ Girl
    - ☐ Boy
    - ☐ Either

10. Would you consider twins?
    - ☐ Yes
    - ☐ No

11. Do you feel you are stable in your relationship as a couple without having children?

_____

_____

_____

_____

_____

_____

_____

12. Which friends and family members would you want to tell about your adoption plans? Which would be supportive and which would not?

_____

_____

_____

_____

_____

_____

_____

13. What level of openness are you willing to consider with birthparents?

    ☐   Completely open adoption

    ☐   Open adoption with reasonable boundaries

    ☐   Exchanging letters and photos only

    ☐   Completely confidential adoption

14. Would you be willing to comply with specific birth family requests regarding child rearing (such as religious instruction, name or schooling)?

    ☐ Yes

    ☐ No

15. Where would you be willing to go to adopt? (Select all that apply)

    ☐ Only in our state

    ☐ Neighboring states

    ☐ Anywhere in US

    ☐ International

16. How much time will you take off work during and after the adoption?

_____

_____

_____

_____

_____

_____

_____

_____

17. How much money would you be willing to spend on an adoption?

18. How much economic hardship would that cause?

19. When and how do you feel children should be told they're adopted?

    ☐ As early as possible / preschool
    ☐ Mid- to late-childhood
    ☐ As adults
    ☐ Only when they ask
    ☐ Only when they find out
    ☐ Never
    ☐ Not sure

20. Would you support/assist your child if he/she wanted to find, contact or have a relationship with his/her birthparents?

    ☐ Yes
    ☐ No
    ☐ Don't know

21. Many adoptive parents have 'dry runs' before they actually adopt. How would you handle an adoption that matched with you but did not end up placing?

    _____
    _____
    _____
    _____
    _____

_____

_____

22. Will you or your spouse (partner) change your workload outside the home after the adoption?

　　　☐　　Yes, I will stay at home with the child

　　　☐　　Yes, my spouse will stay at home with the child

　　　☐　　I will reduce my work load to part time

　　　☐　　My spouse will reduce his/her work load to part time

　　　☐　　Will remain the same

　　　☐　　Already stay-at-home

23. What do you feel you could contribute to a child?

_____

_____

_____

_____

_____

_____

_____

24. What aspects of childrearing are so important to you that you would find it difficult to compromise (such as discipline, religion, schooling, stay-at-home parenting, etc.)?

_____

_____

_____

_____

_____

_____

_____

_____

25. Are you ready to love an adopted child as much as one you gave birth to biologically?

    ☐   Yes
    ☐   No
    ☐   I think so
    ☐   I don't know

26. Would you prefer to continue with infertility treatment before seriously pursuing adoption? If so, why?

_____

_____

_____

_____

_____

_____

_____

27. Deep down do you feel like you are being forced to adopt if you want to have children, adoption as a means to build a family is "second best," or that adoption is your "last resort" if you want to be able to have children?

    (If you answered yes to any of these points, there is a very good chance that you have some significant unresolved issues relating to infertility that you might find beneficial to address and resolve prior to adopting.)

    _____

    _____

    _____

    _____

    _____

    _____

28. What is the ideal adoption situation for you?

29. Ideally, how many children would you like?

_____

_____

_____

30. How long are you willing to wait to adopt?

☐ Up to six months

☐ Six months to 1 year

☐ 1 year to 2 years

☐ 2 to 3 years

☐ However long it takes

c) Fostering

If you are considering fostering a child, review the questions below:

1. Do you have a strong support system of friends and/or family?

_____

_____

_____

_____

_____

2. Are you a patient person?

3. What are your expectations? Not only from the child, but from his or her parents, the state and the fostering experience itself?

4. Do you feel capable to manage the issues and feelings that may be triggered, both in the child and in you, especially if the child has been victimized?

5. Are you willing to have social workers in your home, sometimes every month? Can you work in a partnership with a team of professionals to help the child either get back home or to another permanent placement, such as adoption?

6. Can you envision saying goodbye to a child with whom you've shared so much?

7. What ages of children would you be willing to parent at this time?

8. Do you have a lot of love to give? Are you ready to throw a child his/her first birthday party? Can you help him or her decorate a first Christmas tree or carve a first pumpkin? Help the child to see that families are a great place to grow up and show him/her an excellent role model of healthy family relationships? Give him/her an opportunity to heal and grow?

_____

_____

If you can say "yes" to most of these questions, then <u>call your state foster care representative</u>. You have an excellent chance of being a wonderful foster parent!

d) Living and Loving Child-Free

If you have moved through this process methodically and have now come to the conclusion that your life as a couple will not include raising children together, you may want to create a ritual or visualization that will help you continue to move forward, *together*.

Select a comfortable location that you both enjoy and that holds positive associations and memories for you.

Find a relaxing place to sit or recline. If you are able to do so comfortably, join hands for this exercise.

Allow yourself to breathe deeply in, and let your eyes close as you exhale.

Imagine stepping into a cloud together. Feel the comforting embrace of the cloud and know that you are both safe and secure. As you move through this cloud, feel time and space pass you by. As the cloud disappears, see ahead a place that you both enjoy visiting.

In that moment, experience the depth of love you and your partner share. Observe the joy in each other's eyes. Know how deeply you care for one another.

As you breathe in, use your mind's voice to say, "I am perfect, whole and complete."

Breathe in deeply again, and say to one another, "We are perfect, whole and complete."

Breathe in again, and as you exhale allow your eyes to flutter open. Breathe in all that surrounds you. Drink in your partner and relish in all that your partner brings to the relationship.

Know that you are perfect, whole and complete. You need no one more to comprise the perfect family.

Be well.

Made in the USA
Lexington, KY
30 April 2016